"For married couples facing dilemmas of ... blueprint for growing more personally c... more, and reconnecting with the realm of sensual and sexual pleasure."
—Gina Ogden, PhD, LMFT, author of
The Return of Desire: Rediscovering Your Sexual Passion

"I have read many books on this common problem. Rarely does one come along that's as good as *Wanting Sex Again*. This book is beyond helpful. It works on so many different levels that I would recommend it for anyone in a long-term relationship whether they are having desire problems or not. I can't recommend it highly enough."
—Paul Joannides, PsyD, author of *Guide to Getting It On*

"This book challenges women to not passively accept low desire but rather to identify possible barriers preventing them from experiencing their innate femininity with all its mysterious pleasure."
—Deborah C. Neel, PhD, Licensed Psychologist and Certified Sex Therapist

"Low libido is a difficult, bedeviling problem for many women and couples. Laurie Watson has helped many women recover lost libido, and her book will help many more. Two thumbs up!"
—Michael Castleman, author of *Great Sex*

"Laurie Watson has a gift for relating to women."
—Julie R. McQueen, CHES, Oncology Patient Navigator,
Duke Cancer Center, Raleigh

"A valuable therapeutic resource."
—Carol Casper Figuers, PT, EdD, Associate Professor,
Doctor of Physical Therapy Division, Department of Community and
Family Medicine, Duke University School of Medicine

"Laurie Watson has a wonderful method . . . Her warmth, caring and passion for what she does really shines through."
—Ingrid Harm-Ernandes PT, WCS, BCIA-PMDB,
Orthopedic/Women's Health Specialties, Duke Hospital

"This insightful book is a compass that guides women back to their lost libido. Laurie's message, rich in experience, inspires us to reconnect with our partners and ourselves."
—Polly Watson, MD, FACOG, NCMP, Boylen Healthcare, Raleigh

Wanting Sex Again

HOW TO REDISCOVER
YOUR DESIRE AND HEAL A
SEXLESS MARRIAGE

Laurie J. Watson

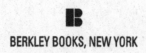

BERKLEY BOOKS, NEW YORK

BERKLEY BOOKS
Published by the Penguin Group
Penguin Group (USA) Inc.
375 Hudson Street, New York, New York 10014, USA
Penguin Group (Canada), 90 Eglinton Avenue East, Suite 700, Toronto, Ontario M4P 2Y3, Canada
(a division of Pearson Penguin Canada Inc.) • Penguin Books Ltd., 80 Strand, London WC2R 0RL,
England • Penguin Group Ireland, 25 St. Stephen's Green, Dublin 2, Ireland (a division of Penguin
Books Ltd.) • Penguin Group (Australia), 250 Camberwell Road, Camberwell, Victoria 3124, Australia
(a division of Pearson Australia Group Pty. Ltd.) • Penguin Books India Pvt. Ltd., 11 Community
Centre, Panchsheel Park, New Delhi—110 017, India • Penguin Group (NZ), 67 Apollo Drive,
Rosedale, Auckland 0632, New Zealand (a division of Pearson New Zealand Ltd.) • Penguin Books
(South Africa) (Pty.) Ltd., 24 Sturdee Avenue, Rosebank, Johannesburg 2196, South Africa

Penguin Books Ltd., Registered Offices: 80 Strand, London WC2R 0RL, England

This book is an original publication of The Berkley Publishing Group.

Every effort has been made to ensure that the information contained in this book is complete and
accurate. However, neither the publisher nor the author is engaged in rendering professional advice
or services to the individual reader. The ideas, procedures, and suggestions contained in this book are
not intended as a substitute for consulting with your physician. All matters regarding your health
require medical supervision. Neither the author nor the publisher shall be liable or responsible for
any loss or damage allegedly arising from any information or suggestion in this book.

While the author has made every effort to provide accurate telephone numbers and Internet addresses
at the time of publication, neither the publisher nor the author assumes any responsibility for errors,
or for changes that occur after publication. Further, the publisher does not have any control over and
does not assume any responsibility for author or third-party websites or their content.

PUBLISHING HISTORY
Berkley trade paperback edition / December 2012

Library of Congress Cataloging-in-Publication Data

Watson, Laurie J.
Wanting sex again : how to rediscover your desire and heal a sexless marriage /
Laurie J. Watson.—1st ed.
p. cm.
Includes bibliographical references.
ISBN 978-0-425-25714-2
1. Marriage. 2. Sex. 3. Man-woman relationships. I. Title.
HQ734.W38 2012
306.81—dc23
2012029575

PRINTED IN THE UNITED STATES OF AMERICA

10 9 8 7 6 5 4 3 2 1

For Derek

· ACKNOWLEDGMENTS ·

I am honored that you've told me your secret fantasies, worst fears, wildest hopes and sacred details of your relationships and sex lives. With gratitude, I acknowledge my many clients for all you've taught me.

I'd like to thank Denise Silvestro and the team (Meredith Giordan, Martin Karlow, and Melissa Broder) at Berkley for believing that women with low libido needed a soft voice to help them. Your painstaking polishing of the manuscript gave the book clarity and crispness. I'm grateful to be working with such an enthusiastic, experienced, and respected publishing house.

My agent, Stephany Evans, with FinePrint Literary Management—you've been a huge champion, not just for my writing but for my career. Your initial call on my birthday was my best-ever present. Thank you!

For all you've taught me in your own writing and in practice and for your generous endorsement of my book, I am humbled. Thanking Michael Castleman, Gina Ogden, Paul Joannides, and Debbie Neel!

With deep gratitude to Susan Perry, my first editor, my endless cheerleader. Your long hours of discussion, revision, teaching, and editing gave birth to this book and to a writer.

Terry Carter for scrupulously advising on commas and content using your long editing experience (and all your vacation days)—thank you. I am proud you think the book will change the lives of women. I would be adrift in the world without your thirty-seven years of friendship.

Thanking Reed Watson for his sharp editing, last-minute, late-night research, and thoughtful, youthful, compassionate commentary on female sexual problems.

I'd like to thank my early encouragers: Sue Weems, who said *write the book!* when I hesitated, my cousin Steve Irvine who thought I could write the book fifteen years ago, Tom and Ilse Mann, salt of the earth, Joy Irvine Garratt, my cousin and experienced publicist—you made platform development sound easy and possible. Your support both professionally and personally has been a blessing.

I am indebted to Dr. Polly Watson for hours of her time, editing and sharing research on menopause and vulvar pain problems, Dr. John Marks for generously teaching me about the anatomy and physiology of vulvar pain, and Dr. Myra Teasley for her expertise on menopause and her constant encouragement. For the many physicians in Wake County who trusted me with their patients when I opened the practice in Raleigh, I am grateful.

Thanks to readers of the manuscript for their editing and commentary: Peggy Payne, Meg McHenry, Nance Murphy, Clare Stadlen, Carrie Roberson, Susan Rountree, Melanie Jones, and Joe Dew.

Many mentors, teachers and therapists have added to my understanding of sexual functioning, human development and relationships. Thanking the AASECT listserve (A-club), Dr. Ernie Braasch, Rebecca Dnistran, Christine Erskine, Jeff Levy, Dr. Linda Norris, Dr. Wanda Radford, Dr. Dave Rice, Dr. Jill Scharff, Dr. Alan Stern, and Dr. Jeanne Yorke.

I am furthermore thankful for Christy Warner; your handling of all the details of my professional life keep me from being lost, disorganized, and unhappy.

For Wednesday school participants: Kathie and David Henry, Kim and Jim McGimsey, Carol and Gene Walker, and my dear friend Natalie Jacobs Chigozie—your stabilizing love, insight and endless support have kept my own relationship going. Thank you.

For my mom, Dottie Irvine, who could not wait to tell her little girl about the wonders of sex.

My sons, Reed, Soren, and Tristan for also believing that this book was worth the sacrifice of their mother's time for years on end. Hoping this book makes the world a better place for you.

For my husband, Derek—you were right; I could write a book. My utmost gratitude for all the creature comforts you brought me while writing, for taking over with the boys while I was busy, for wanting to listen to me, and for spurring me on. For your friendship and love, I am yours. Again and again, with you.

· CONTENTS ·

You're Not the Only One

"I never want to have sex again!" blurted out Karen, a thirty-three-year-old willowy blonde dressed in pinstripes, within two minutes of walking into my office. I wasn't surprised, really. I hear this sentiment nearly every day from women calling to make an appointment.

As a sex therapist and marital counselor, I know that a heartbreaking lack of sexual desire happens in the bedrooms of even the most apparently solid marriages.

"I don't want you to think I have a bad marriage," Karen went on to say that day. "Sex is the only thing we ever fight about." She couldn't quite look me in the eye yet. Talking about your own sex life isn't easy.

Like most women, when her libido slipped to the vanishing point, Karen first turned to her gynecologist. Sex is a bodily function and doctors take care of bodies, so that all makes sense. Then the doctor gives a reference to a therapist and we worry that our heads are screwed up.

But you are not crazy; many women struggle with low sexual desire and there are many causes. This book is about figuring out how you can want sex again.

Overwhelmed by Life, Underwhelmed by Sex

Having an orgasm may simply not be high on our to-do list, considering the demands of work, kids, and for many of us, ailing parents. Most of the time we feel lucky to have a moment to breathe freely at the end of a busy day. Don't men see all the chores that need to be done? We're enraged at our husband's oblivion. We chafe at the idea of undressing for someone who isn't pulling his fair share. Resentment has become a monster under the bed.

Like Karen, we've heard our neighbors joke about their husbands pestering them for more sex, but in our marriage no one's laughing. In fact, the tension and anger flowing out of the bedroom have reached the point where we're getting concerned that the kids might be affected.

Messages from our childhood about sex include "don't" and silence. Remembering every time Daddy went to slip his arms around Mommy's waist, we can still see her roll her eyes and sigh. When we asked Mom about sex, she avoided our question simply saying, "Good girls don't." And when we did overhear our mother talk about sex with friends, it was in whispers and with more than a hint of disgust. Helplessly, we hear ourselves sound more like our mother every day and we'd swear our husband is mutating into our father before our very eyes. Worse, we're terrified that our situation is unique—dysfunctional.

While we haven't been begging for sex, we have begged for romance. "Surprise me! Seduce me!" we've cried. Okay, maybe we haven't been as vocal as we should be, but we're tired of asking for what we need to make us feel "in the mood." He used to be creative when we dated, but now heaven forbid he'd think to call a sitter so we can go out for a romantic evening.

Come to think of it, he's never been a good kisser, and how do you talk about that? If he bumps us one more time with an erection when we're at the stove, we just might throw the spatula. And when did he get the idea that groping was foreplay?

Overburdened women are often depressed about their circumstances, let alone their intimacy quotient. Sometimes, the medication that lifts depression also kills our drive and mutes our orgasms. So sex suffers either way: be happier on meds and feel dead "down there," or be miserable because you can't get out of bed much less want to get back in.

Culture's Messages

It certainly doesn't help that we're surrounded by images of nubile models and actresses in the media implying that everyone else is having wild, passionate sex with no difficulty at all. Every time we pick up groceries, *Cosmopolitan* screams at us to care about "His G-spot and 7 Other Moan Spots," and we don't even know how to find our own (or if it matters).

Feeling sexy is damn hard because our culture despises real women's bodies. With shows like *America's Next Top Model* and Victoria's Secret lingerie commercials, we don't even like changing our socks if our husband's in the room. Maybe we haven't had sex above the covers since the children were born. And don't anyone dare leave a light on—a sheet could slip away and a cellulite dimple show!

Day in and day out, we are sent double messages: look sexy but don't actually be sexual. All of our young life we were told girls who wanted it warranted ugly names. Nice girls sit with their legs or ankles crossed. Good girls are modest and chaste. This programming has become ingrained in our subconscious. Now our husband is upset when we're still following the good-girl rules and won't tell him the grand old secret: how we like to be touched so that we will enjoy sex and actually *want* to be sexual.

Later in life, we come to fear the image of the hag; we're pounded by the message that aging isn't sexy. Maybe we're afraid our husband is having an affair with that sexy, young assistant from his office who we watched suspiciously at last year's holiday party. Our ego takes another hit. Or we get hot flashes and night sweats and we swear to our doctors that the marriage is fine but our body really feels different. We've been told to get on hormone replacement therapy for our bones; we've been told to get off it for our breasts. With so many medical breakthroughs recently, can't someone make a pill that will make us shiver for our spouse again? Where's our Viagra?

What Happened to Us?

We may finally ask, "Is it so wrong to want sex less than my husband? Maybe he has unrealistic expectations. Maybe it's like licorice liqueur. I enjoy it every once in a while, but I don't want it as a routine nightcap—it's too intense. I don't think I'd even want it once a week. So what? Why am I the 'wrong' one?" We're tired of being blamed for all the marital problems.

Frustratingly, our bodies used to go crazy with desire. We remember feeling excited about seeing some guy at a party and feeling giddy inside. That first touch sent electric shocks and we got wet. Making love turned us inside out. When did hot turn to ho-hum?

Female bodies are built for sex. We are the love machines! Only women can have multiple orgasms. Only our bodies have an organ—the clitoris—devoted exclusively to pleasure. What men can do fast, we can do better. Our capacity for orgasm begins in the womb and, unless severely interrupted by disease or accident, doesn't end until the grave. While desire is easily upended, orgasmic functioning usually works like a dream, given enough time and foreplay. Some of us can even have orgasms just by thinking about sex—without any physical contact.

So what's wrong with us? Why aren't we interested in sex anymore? Can we get desire back?

Men's desire is constant, through tiredness, through arguments, through baby screams, through indigestion, through middle age, and through rain and sleet because of the huge amount of testosterone, which can be three hundred times more than the amount that our bodies produce. We'd love to have our bodies push us for sex. In fact, this is the most common reason women say they have no libido. We don't always have the same biological prompt—a sexual urge, an instinctual nudge, or an outright horny feeling. A woman with low desire is like a Porsche with a tank full of gas and a broken starter.

Sundry Other Problems

Poor sexual education or unrealistic expectations between a woman and her husband lead to quite a bit of unhappiness. But fortunately these are quickly remedied, and couples usually experience a vastly improved sex life within a few sessions of counseling. Learning to have orgasms, developing a mutually explicit and erotic language, perfecting technique, and deciding what sexual acts are mutually pleasurable and acceptable take minimal coaching. Sometimes a woman schedules only one therapy session to ask a question and gain reassurance about whether she is sexually normal; that may be all the help she needs. The first few chapters of this book tackle those less complex issues.

Most sexual concerns stem from an interpersonal struggle in the marriage. The bind in mid-marriage (after the honeymoon until the kids graduate high school or twelve to twenty years in) becomes a constant tug-of-war between being too close and being too distant from each other. With or without children, all couples need both autonomy and closeness. Unfortunately, sex is often caught in the strained rope between these needs. In the next set of chapters (the second tier of complexity), we'll examine these seemingly opposing needs as a couple becomes a family. We'll discuss motherhood juxtaposed on the erotic self. As our family of origin plays an enormous role in our sexual self, several chapters point out how old legacies struggle to stay alive and how they interrupt our personal and sexual flexibility and joy.

We'll see how seduction and initiation serve as a micro-battleground for the relational struggles. We'll look at how, for optimal personal and partner growth, women crave a sense of relatedness in order to have continued desire, and how we can use our minds to sustain libido with fantasy.

The specific issue of physical pain during sex deserves a chapter of its own, as many women suffer silently and feel ashamed when their doctors tell them it's all in their heads. The meaning and devastation of an affair from the betrayed partner's vantage point will be examined, as well as the couple's potential for a reconstruction of the sexual and marital bond. Another chapter examines childhood sexual trauma and its role in shutting down a survivor's sex drive.

Lastly we'll consider how our partner's difficulties contribute to our own, how menopause and the image of the crone impacts our own self-image. A communication technique is offered for resolving volatile problems. Finally, we'll examine the dilemma of knowing when low desire does signify love is lost for good. Sometimes these latter problems can take considerable time to change, and need additional professional expertise from physicians and physical therapists. At times, personal healing can come only through ending the partnership or marriage.

There's Help

People in conflicted relationships usually begin by trying to talk to each other, but sometimes that only seems to worsen matters between them. They can see the trees (the problems they're having) but not the forest (the core issues). It's dark and hopeless and every time they try to get out of the woods they find themselves wandering in a circle, back to the same place. Yet after focusing on sexual problems in my practice for so long, I often see from my bird's-eye view that even with repetitive patterns, there's a path out to greater happiness and sexual satisfaction. That trail, hidden to the couple before, leads to a strong, true, inner erotic self for her and deep connection emotionally and sexually with each other. When both spouses work together on these issues, it's most effective, but even one partner alone can change her role and see real improvement.

At any age, the mystery of female lust doesn't reside in the body alone or merely in our chemistry. Balancing our hormones perfectly doesn't guarantee the revival of feelings because sex is bigger than our bodies. Desire is inextricably tangled in our minds, our memories, our fantasies, our upbringing, our relationships, our shame, our exaltation, our connection to our partner, as well as the breathing space between us.

In each chapter, we'll peek into the lives of women and couples and listen to their stories. You, as a reader, will be able to recognize parts of yourself and locate your concerns in the various sex therapy sessions. Although all of the people profiled are composites, they are based on real people and real stories I've encountered in my practice. All names and identifying details have been changed. I am indebted to my clients for what they have taught me about sexuality and long-term relationship through their courage and vulnerability. While a woman may feel that it's all her fault because she's the one without desire, nearly all problems with sexual intimacy involve issues brought by both partners. And although you may feel like this is an insurmountable problem, I have never sat with a woman or a couple and not felt hopeful about finding a solution to her low desire and its roots. The actions necessary to change aren't always easy. The choices we have to make to get the desire back can be tough. If the answer were as simple as new lingerie or a magic technique, you wouldn't be reading this book. The hardest thing about changing your sex life is that it usually means changing yourself. But joyful, meaningful, erotic sex can be—and is meant to be—yours.

Help Yourself

Make the ideas in this chapter your own by reflecting on and responding to the following questions:

1. What would life be like if the whole conflict over sex could somehow be removed from your relationship?

2. What are your concerns about your sex life?

3. What obstacles do you already know get in the way of your eroticism?

4. How has sex changed over the course of your relationship?

CHAPTER ONE

Wedding Cake and Other Anti-Aphrodisiacs: Early Marital Problems

In the unadorned conference room of a pretty church favored for weddings, I taught premarital classes to couples for seven years. Most of these men and women were young; all were misty-eyed with romance, buzzing with wedding plans and limitless optimism. When I brought up the issue of sexual problems, nudges and covert glances passed between them, as if to say, "Sexual problems? They'll never happen to us because clearly we're the most sexually compatible couple on the planet!"

Couples in the earliest days of love simply don't want to believe that everyone has sexual difficulties at some point.

In fact, early marriage is rife with sexual problems. Who knew? After all, we don't have any idea what goes on in other people's bedrooms. Sex usually happens—and stays—in the dark, literally. Yet some of the couples from my premarital classes would turn up later admitting that something had gone wrong. Even couples who don't formalize their love with a ceremony usually find themselves with similar difficulties within two years.

Six erotic tasks accomplished in early marriage set a foundation for strong and vibrant intimacy throughout the years. When Karen from our introduction—married just a year—persuaded her husband to come to her second appointment, I had them begin thinking about the "who, what, where, when, why, and how" brass tacks of adjustment.

What Went Wrong?

Both dressed casually in after-work jeans and relaxed T-shirts. I saw that Karen had accurately described just how dreamy her husband was. His strained grin told me he might feel anxious about meeting a sex therapist.

"My husband is a great guy," Karen had told me at the initial session a week before. "He's the love of my life. He's handsome and intelligent and all I've ever wanted in a man. He listens to me. He gets me. The way I feel about him makes me question my sanity about what I'm going to say next. I don't want to have sex with him . . . I don't want to have sex at all. From the time we moved in together, it's like someone walked into my head and flipped off the switch marked 'Sex Drive.' It's not his fault. In fact, he is the best lover I've ever been with. Now, I'm shaking his confidence. He's started asking me if I find him attractive or if I really want to be married! Every conversation we have about sex seems to split us apart further."

Shortly after their wedding, Karen's job responsibilities had increased, and she noticed a correlating drop in her desire to have sex. Now, with my prompting, Simon filled in his version of events.

"I feel pretty dejected. I really love Karen, and sex was good right from the start. She's more tired now because, with the recession, she's had to cover two additional states for her sales territory. I can understand that, and I'm grateful she survived her company's layoffs. But I don't know if I can keep going under all the stress I've got too, without sex to help me get through it. And I really don't get it. Our sex life just went 'poof!' as soon as we married."

Karen looked as though she were going to interrupt here, but I indicated that she ought to let Simon finish his summary.

"Sure," he went on, "there's probably a third less time on weeknights now compared with before. But it's like her desire dropped by three hundred percent. Do you know the old joke about certain foods being anti-aphrodisiacs? Well, in our case, wedding cake sure did the trick."

Honeymoon Blues

Weddings, strangely, are often followed by downshifts in erotic lovemaking. Unconscious shifts in intimacy, power struggles, and repetition of old themes from our childhood are often to blame. But Karen and Simon seemed to be having some basic trouble with the various aspects of sexual adjustment. Unfortunately, what begins as the need for clarification can, if unresolved, result in years of lockdown and misunderstandings.

After Simon spoke, Karen shared her perspective. "I think the lack of time has impacted us quite a bit. We don't luxuriate in lovemaking anymore. Simon used to spend hours trying to get in my pants when we first dated, and he'd try everything. I loved the chase; it was exciting. Now there's this expectation that we'll just do it most nights."

"Wow!" Simon whipped his head around to face her. "Sweetheart, the chase has been replaced by a new game. I ask and you say no. I was doing you a favor by keeping it short and sweet. You never want sex. Even when I try to go down on you, you resist."

"I wanted sex in Cancún and you were the one who turned me down," Karen retorted petulantly.

"Cancún!" He turned to face me and explained. "We were on our honeymoon and I got the flu! Seriously, it lasted three days and I thought I'd die. Yes, I turned her down and it was on our honeymoon, but for Pete's sake, there was nothing I could do about it. She brings it up all the time as if that sole rejection is her excuse to never initiate again. It was like some sort of capital offense."

More tension filled the room than Karen had hinted at in our initial session. Young couples can be afraid of arguments and thus avoid the important airing of differences, which might lead to greater understanding. Part of the bubble of new love is the misconception that the two are soul mates, emotional twins. The sudden bursting of this illusion often causes either the husband or the wife—or both—to begin fearing that they chose the wrong mate. Deep down, whether they're aware of it or not, they long for a symbiotic ideal where their spouse can read their mind. So often we think true love means a person knows what we need before we ask. But mature love means more separateness and acknowledgment that no one can really know our needs unless we make them plain.

But the good news is that the friction of sexual negotiations in the early married phase brings to life the very distinctions between husband and wife that will keep the sparks going. Without a certain level of conflict and subsequent discussion, sex suffers as each partner's silent expectations come between them and, brick by brick, begin to separate them.

Erotic Task #1: Negotiate an acceptable balance of who initiates sexual encounters.

In an egalitarian relationship, there may seem to be only one right answer to who should initiate: take turns. Simon had fantasies that Karen's aggressiveness in their early dating days would continue. He dreamed of her arriving at his office in the old trench-coat-with-nothing-on-underneath.

Karen protested, "I never really did more than smile at Simon or put my hand on his thigh. I guess that was initiation, but he still made the first move. I don't know where he got the idea that I was some exhibitionist."

"A trench coat opened in the privacy of my office hardly makes you an exhibitionist, Karen," Simon replied with a pout. "And trust me, that is one of my mildest fantasies."

Actually, Karen did feel sexy and occasionally had thoughts about making love, but they were doused if Simon appeared uninterested. Getting ready for bed, she'd wonder if he was going to initiate. When he was engrossed in TV and didn't glance up, she'd climb into bed feeling hurt that he hadn't found her more interesting than his show. Every time she felt disappointed, she dialed down her feelings of desire just a little more.

Men were supposed to initiate, according to her inner rules.

Having to be suggestive now might mean Simon didn't find her attractive enough to be perpetually turned on. It didn't occur to her that seduction was a two-way street.

Even though Simon initiated far more than she accepted, these nagging feelings of rejection were like poisoned darts in Karen's heart, causing her to shut down. For her, the honeymoon rejection felt like a catastrophe. It held an unfounded significance for her, but she couldn't shake the feeling. It was perfectly understandable—even to Karen, on some level—that Simon, suffering from nausea and vomiting, would not want to have sex, but Karen couldn't help how she felt.

It's not a surprise that this honeymoon mishap resulted in injuries that were disproportional to the "offense." Because the honeymoon symbolizes sexual paradise for a new couple, even small problems can seem like their future is ruined. Much of the trouble this couple was having seemed to be the mismatch of her fantasy of a strong, romantic, new husband on moonlight-drenched beaches juxtaposed with the gritty picture of her weak, feverish husband throwing up in the bathroom of their hotel room. His turndown happened just as he was getting sick, and what she recalled was the humiliation of being in a negligee and asking him to come onto the terrace and his preferring to crawl into bed alone. Now Karen worried that if she initiated sex, she'd be turned down again.

Initiation doesn't have to be completely fifty-fifty if couples can work out an understanding that who starts is less important than that the experience itself be pleasurable and restorative. During some stages of marriage, especially the child-rearing years, couples can learn to make use of the husband's bountiful testosterone, which results in natural and spontaneous initiation. A woman can learn to "borrow" her husband's testosterone, if he will initiate and she practices more of what sex researcher Dr. Rosemary Basson describes as "triggered desire," which is the willingness to engage in sexual activity as opposed to spontaneous craving for sex.[1] Her husband can be the one to express overt desire more frequently and to take responsibility for the bulk of initiation. But because everyone wants to feel sexually desirable, men also need to have reassuring expressions of sexual interest. Women must learn to accept the risks of initiation so that sex happens when they are at their day's or cycle's height of desire (I'll discuss both of these some more later in the book), rather than always relying on a chance synchronicity.

Time for Bed (and Sex), Honey

Simon continued to describe their predicament. "Okay, so maybe she didn't actually initiate as aggressively as I imagined she had, but I want her to want me like she did before. I don't want her just to have sex because I want to—I want her to want to do it too."

Karen quickly seconded the idea. "That's the way I want it too! I didn't turn my desire off on purpose! This is radically different from when we met for me too, and I hate it!"

She described how Simon usually initiated. He'd wait until bedtime and then reach for her in the dark under the blankets. Furthermore, Simon thought "couples should go to bed at the same time," but didn't take into account that Karen had to get up earlier than he did.

"So I end up waiting for him to be ready for bed because he's got one more show to watch or one more thing to do. And I'm a little mad because I don't think he takes me into consideration regarding the time. And yeah, by then I'm closed off. If I say yes to sex, it's another half hour before I can go to sleep, and if I say no, I feel so guilty that it takes me a half hour anyway before I can fall asleep."

"Tell us how you'd like him to initiate," I prompted her.

"I'd like him to tell me he wants *me*. He used to say romantic things, look at me, and put a little effort into it."

Two problems were represented here. Karen liked a verbal suggestion about sex. She wanted Simon to flirt and compliment her. When they dated, he had been full of sexual innuendo, and now their evening conversations centered around taking care of the business of life. When Simon reached for her in bed, it felt presumptuous and impersonal.

Second, the timing of sex—bedtime itself—was too late for her. Yet she had never let him know the full extent of her growing resentment. In session, I coached Karen to speak up on both counts. She also needed to argue that going to sleep when it was appropriate for her own needs would actually give her much-needed energy for their intimate life. Her acquiescence to his belief about mutual bedtimes was sabotaging their sex life.

Simon said, "I think I'm delaying the bedtime hoping for some signal from Karen that she wants to be with me. I'm afraid if I ask she'll just say no. By the time we're under the covers, I'm desperate. It's frustrating to be hearing this for the first time. I wish Karen would have told me what she was feeling. I can go to bed earlier; it just feels empty to go to bed knowing the day is over without connecting.

Erotic Task #2: Agree on how sex is to be initiated.

How we initiate can predetermine the outcome of a sexual encounter. Some individuals like a verbal approach and will use words to ask for sex (or will want their partner to use words). Others prefer to be caressed and sexually "taken" the way it's done in the movies. To Karen, Simon's end-of-the-day routine felt like she was his sleeping pill.

Karen yearned for masterful verbal seduction. She'd read Harlequin romance novels during her adolescence and fantasized about someone sweeping her off her feet with clever, sexy dialogue that made her ache with arousal. Earlier dates with Simon approximated her fantasies, like a trip they took up the coast and an apparent spontaneous overnight in a theme hotel for lovers. As it turned out, Simon had planned the excursion for weeks but pulled it off as an impulsive trip. His thoughtfulness made her feel special. His banter had held a sexual edge that turned her on.

But now his reach for her under the covers seemed rote, like mechanical need. Gone was the conversation. Gone was the wine and romance during the evening. The change from the chase of courtship to regular married sex disappointed Karen. She felt less valuable to Simon because he no longer put any effort into seduction.

And yet it never occurred to Simon that his wife was feeling taken for granted. He was flummoxed because, for him, married sex was supposed to be the equivalent of permanently winning at Candy Land. He had unlimited viewing access to his wife's goodies every morning when she showered and dressed. She was in his bed every night tantalizing him with her nearness. He loved rolling over in the middle of the night and feeling the warmth of her body. Marital sex was a hard-won prize and he meant to revel in it. And he was delighted at the thought of being taken for granted in bed. He expected marriage to mean regular, perhaps nightly, sex.

Certainly, some of Karen's expectations needed to be modified, while the more feasible ones could be communicated in order to give Simon a fighting chance to fulfill them. She also needed to bring some of the missing aspects she craved to the table, or in this case, to the bed. She needed to verbally flirt with him. However, this was difficult for Karen. Learning to hear and twist conversation to the sexual was challenging for her. She had to fight a critical part of her mind that accused her of no longer being a "nice" woman when she was behaving suggestively. On the other hand, her mate's exultation of the sensual was a beautiful demonstration of how safe he felt in their relationship, and she wanted more of it.

With some help, Karen began to see herself less as a sexual reward for Simon, and more as a participant in intimacy with her own unique cravings. Once Simon rediscovered how his quick wit turned her on, he was able to ramp things up again.

Never (or Always) Before Coffee

When Simon and Karen were dating, they would have sex several times over a weekend, sometimes before they went out, sometimes after dinner, and often in the morning. In reality, they didn't see each other much during the week, and by Friday, their hunger to be in each other's arms dominated all thoughts and activities.

But now Karen's growing resentment turned their weekends into nothing more than a repeat of their difficult weeknight problems. Weekends were time off! She resisted using recreation time to do anything that seemed to encroach further on her personal space. As we'll see more clearly a bit later, too much closeness in early marriage can have its own impact on libido.

Erotic Task #3: Consider each mate's preference for when to make love.

Some people sing with energy in the early morning and others can't pry their eyes open until two cups of coffee past ten o'clock. It's good to take advantage of natural peak times. But many couples complain that he's a morning person and she's an evening person and day never meets night. This is actually a manifestation of a power struggle, as there are always weekends or occasional times in between when both partners are awake and energized. I know that my clients can organize their lives to get together for at least one hour a week for a counseling session, and so, objectively, the timing argument becomes moot. In fact, I will say to couples, "Take the money, take the hour, and rent a hotel room before you consult a therapist. See if that doesn't resolve many of the problems." For example, one couple insisted that timing was the primary barrier that kept them apart. Yet they both worked from home via the Internet. They acted stunned when I suggested a noontime rendezvous.

But You Used to Like That!

Simon had alluded to another frustration earlier in our conversation: he would like to give Karen oral sex but she resisted it. According to Karen, the extra fifteen minutes required to take a shower wasn't worth it. "Yeah, I used to let him do that, but now I'd just rather get it over with."

Simon wasn't crazy about her response. "Great! Just great! Yeah, let's get it over with! Is that how you feel? I thought you liked me licking you and it seemed like that's the only way you could come."

"It is the only way I come. And I'm not coming very much, if you've noticed," Karen tossed back.

Simon was confused and frustrated by Karen's comments. "I try to do you, you resist, and now you complain about it."

Karen tried to explain in more detail, making an effort to keep the defeated tone out of her voice. She didn't like oral sex on a quickie night, as she wasn't ready for it. In fact, none of their nights felt long enough for her to relax and enjoy oral sex. Karen needed to have orgasms to maintain desire—the whole episode seemed pointless otherwise—and she wasn't having very many. Their techniques for making love, especially oral sex, that had worked reliably before, were being pushed aside—by her. Indeed, something very confusing was going on here.

Erotic Task #4: Make expectations explicit about what sex will be like and which acts are going to happen on any given day.

Couples need to communicate whether they are going to have a sensual time of massage and luxurious lovemaking, a romantic and interactive interlude, an acting out of erotic fantasies, a utilitarian quickie, a fast and furious tumble, mutual masturbation, or sixty-nine (i.e., simultaneous oral sex). When two people have been making love with each other for a long time, they develop a shorthand for these expectations and can more easily read each other. New lovers must be patient about learning each other's style.

Karen and Simon were often a half step off, with her desiring long, slow lovemaking but feeling they didn't have the time, and him wanting her so desperately that he tried to get in a quickie whenever possible. With some compromising, they began to see the different ways they were viewing their weeknight sex. Over the course of therapy, Karen took a pragmatic approach to weeknights. She enjoyed the closeness but dropped her expectations of having an orgasm during a quickie. And if she did decide she wanted one, she pulled out her vibrator. She became more openly demanding on the weekends with clear expectations that they were going to wring the life out of their sheets.

How much variety does each of you like? How much spice do you need to keep from boredom? How much risk do you crave? What one partner finds acceptable and desirable may have to be negotiated against the other's feelings of taboo or revulsion. Risk balanced against comfort prevents sex from becoming stale. Variety doesn't mean that a woman has to do something illegal or, to her mind, immoral. Having sex in the car parked on lovers' lane may seem like taking an unnecessary risk of exposure. But perhaps the same car parked in her own garage would feel safe enough, while still novel and thus exciting.

Risk comes from openly sharing what you think about sex, sharing your private fantasies rather than being about near-public exhibitionism. It's the difference between your spouse sharing what he did that day and how he felt about what he did that day—the first may be informative, but the second is infinitely more intimate. Women worry about never satisfying their husband's need for variety or worry that giving in a little will eventually mean doing things they don't want to do. They don't trust themselves to voice their reservations adequately, so they let their body say it for them and shut down sexual desire. And they sometimes even don't dare to make changes that could be comfortable for them. Easy revelations of what she's fantasizing about, what she'd like to try tonight, what she remembers has really worked before, would offer a vulnerability that would deeply satisfy many husbands.

You're Speaking My Language

When Simon referred to oral sex as "licking," Karen flinched. Their erotic language preferences were getting in the way of their getting connected. His embarrassed her. She explained, "Most of the time Simon is just a funny guy, but when he's talking about sex, he goes too far. He'll say stuff like, 'I liked lickin' your pussy last night.' It's just crass. Then I'll feel humiliated for letting him know I enjoyed it—sort of like he'll lord it over me. And he'll bring it up at breakfast. It's not enough that we had sex the night before—he wants to talk about it some more."

Karen was uncomfortable with the words Simon used when he brought up intimate details afterward. In fact, Simon admitted that her morning standoffishness amused him. He liked watching her blush.

Erotic Task #5: Develop a mutual erotic language.

At the risk of seeming to align with Karen, I said, "Simon, there are plenty of women who like risqué or coarser language. And you obviously like that kind of language. But Karen doesn't, at least not when she's no longer in the throes of passion. It has little to do with low libido, no libido, or high libido. Many women have a modesty barrier that drops when they're aroused, and you're asking her to be uninhibited at a time when she's kind of past that. It sounds like she feels exposed for having shown you her pleasure."

Defending himself, he said, "But for me, that morning recap is part of the fun."

Yes, it was part of his fun, but not hers. She felt too vulnerable the next day for such explicit replay. Did Karen want anything in particular from Simon the morning after, or would she prefer silence?

"No, I don't need silence. But I'm sick of the junior high review and analysis. Why couldn't he just kiss me good morning and say he loves me?"

Wanting to have it all, Simon tried to push further. "I want more freedom between us, though, not less. It would feel like even more restriction to watch my language too."

Rather than reducing his spontaneity or fun, his awareness of how his words affected Karen would help them both. She enjoyed a more sophisticated, clever communication style, and Simon was good at it. But occasionally his word choice grated on her and left her feeling shut down. And that was not his intention! It was within his power to pick terms that would give her more feelings of appreciation and love in the morning. Perhaps in a steamy embrace she would like more explicit words and I asked her to consider this. But in the long run, Simon was losing a lot by having fun at Karen's expense.

Understandably, for many people, talking about lovemaking after the act is enjoyable because it keeps the experience going, but it doesn't generate more sexual feelings if the other person isn't comfortable with it.

Do It Like an Expert—20/20 Style

When each of you knows how to touch the other to bring about the most pleasure, you are communicating intimately. With the utmost tact and discipline, we must learn how to correct subtle touches. Saying "please touch me this way" or "I'd love for you to do that" takes a great deal of courage and vulnerability. Frustrated lovers beg their spouses for a morsel of information so they can improve. Directions should be positive and specific. Lights on and blankets off grant the most accurate access for a man to learn a woman's anatomy, though it can challenge a woman's modesty. But women often tell me that he really has no idea where her clitoris is, and she remains frustrated by his fumbling. Or if he's found it, he thinks that ringing it like a doorbell will open her up for intercourse.

In a highly aroused state, a woman may be ready for intercourse very quickly. Early courting, elaborate dates, risky sexual adventures, or an affair are all unique situations that may induce soaring excitement in the body before one touch occurs. But it's unrealistic for a married or long-term couple to wait to have sex only during special celebrations or in high-risk situations. Ongoing, regular, married lovemaking can reach lusty heights even if most sessions begin with her at a point of simple mental acquiescence. Her motivation may come more from the wish for emotional connection and transform into sexual hunger after she is aroused. Desire follows arousal. Because males usually experience sexual hunger before arousal or nearly simultaneous with arousal, this pattern can be disappointing if it's misinterpreted as lack of attraction or lack of love on the woman's part.

Too much pressure to have every session rock your or your partner's world takes away from the stress-relieving, playful, and love-affirming roles that sex plays in a marriage. Psychiatrist and sex therapist Dr. David Scharff explains in *The Sexual Relationship* that sex functions in a marriage to ease the wear and tear of daily life, reconnect two people in body and soul, and facilitate forgiveness for the daily irritations of living with another. "Good-enough sex," he writes, while not perfect, sometimes meets one's need for sex in exactly the way it is desired.[2] For a woman, this requires a focus on pleasure, a relaxed time frame, and regular orgasms.

The peaks of extraordinary sex spring forth from the foothills of good-enough sex. Without steady, ordinary sex, the odds of having extraordinary encounters are slim. As with anything you want to become expert at, the more you do it, the better the odds you'll have an especially good session.

Erotic Task #6: Master technique.

Time—and enough of it—are the key to arousal for a woman. Desire kicks in once the body feels something. She wants it once she's having it. Transitioning to a sexy mind-set often takes about twenty minutes of slow undressing, full body-to-body contact, intimate sharing, and leisurely caressing. During this seduction phase, many women do not want their genitals touched for physiological reasons. It doesn't feel good. Or it feels dry, sandy, ticklish, painful, or worse—about as sexual as rubbing their elbow. When their genitals are touched before enough arousal has taken place, women often conclude that their body's feedback means it's not their night. Once aroused, a woman may take an average of twenty minutes of direct, nonstop, skillful clitoral stimulation to reach orgasm. The 20/20 solution—twenty minutes of foreplay, twenty minutes of sexual touch—often translates to bountiful desire and orgasm.

Karen had already confided that Simon homed in on her clitoris within minutes of starting sex. Furthermore, she had never bothered to explain to him that oral sex only a couple of minutes into physical contact was too soft and delicate a sensation to spark arousal. She needed a firmer touch to get going. Not finding herself turned on immediately, she would become self-conscious about how long it was taking to respond. Pretty soon that critical voice in her head would make disparaging remarks such as "What's wrong with you? He's probably bored. He can tell you don't like it. You're not much of a sexual hottie." And so on. Feeling like a failure for not getting aroused more quickly only ensured that she wouldn't feel anything.

Even during their hot dating encounters, she felt slightly uncomfortable at the start of their lovemaking unless a little alcohol helped relax her. She'd always loosen up as the night wore on, feeling calmer about the hours ahead. And weeknights were no longer conducive to drinking because she knew she had to get up and be out on the road the next day. She would blame and criticize to cover up her feelings of awkwardness about saying what she liked and how she liked it. So their system of feedback got screwed up. She couldn't say what was wrong; he couldn't fix what he didn't know.

Simon responded with frustration at first. "I try to make it a quickie because I know she's tired and really doesn't want it anyway. I'm more than willing to give her more time. I procrastinate going to bed because it puts off the disappointment of not having sex. I suppose I'm avoiding her 'no.'"

At my suggestion, he committed to one creative date over the weekend that also included an opportunity for relaxed sexual pleasure. He started to tease her when she seemed bored in bed, threatening to stop the pleasure if she got too close to orgasm. Invariably, this turned her watchful anxiety about not getting aroused on its head. Suddenly she was trying not to go over the cliff of orgasm, and she found her arousal intensifying and quickening. Oral sex was offered to her closer to orgasm, when her modesty was long gone. That way, Karen found it, once again, exquisite.

Help Yourself

1. Compare your sexual responses now with earlier in your relationship. What are the two of you doing differently?

2. What were the best and worst sexual moments of your early lovemaking or honeymoon?

3. Name three sexual risks that you haven't taken but would be willing to try.

CHAPTER TWO

Tug-of-War: Getting the Right Closeness/Distance

Wild sex is a great way for a relationship to start, but it's no insurance against waning desire. And once you've experienced intimate ecstasy, a sexual slowdown or a total halt is understandably disturbing. Why does sex fade in so many relationships?

Can it be that plunging libido is merely the inevitable lapse of romance resulting from reordering priorities or yielding to busyness? We know that feeling overworked, overwhelmed, or overtired, does change desire. But there is a central problem in marriage—how to balance our needs for closeness and separateness—that sex gets caught between.

From Hot to Cool

Like Sam and Cheryl, whom we will meet next, many couples are mystified about why they were so sexually compatible in the beginning only to find themselves growing cooler a short while into the marriage. The same electrifying memories that proved their capability to create fireworks now frustrate them. Exhilaration seems to be a fingertip's breadth away, yet tantalizingly out of reach.

Sam, forty-six, sat on my couch looking bitter. Desperate to get their sex life fixed, he had been the one to seek out a sex therapist. He and Cheryl were middle-aged newlyweds. Both had been married before, and had children ranging from middle school to college age. A software engineer, he dressed in a blue button-down dress shirt and khakis. Cheryl, a part-time tax accountant, dressed beautifully, her white short-sleeved, fine mesh-knit top and gray fitted slacks set off by a stunning silver medallion necklace.

Sam had chosen the seat directly in front of me, perhaps to better secure my attention. Cheryl sat on the opposite end of the couch from him, her arms and legs crossed.

Sam's initial statement was spoken angrily. "From our honeymoon forward, Cheryl hasn't wanted to have sex."

Since I had already talked with Sam on the phone, I knew a little about his side of the story. Now I gently asked Cheryl what she felt.

"I feel like he's dragged me in here to publicly shame me for being a failure as a wife," she said, despondence in her voice. "I don't know why I don't want to have sex anymore. I just don't.

Maybe it is all my fault and he should leave me. Sex is all he thinks about and all we ever talk about. No, I should say 'fight about' because we really don't talk anymore."

Asked how long they'd been married, Sam replied, "Two years. Long years." He darted a fuming look toward Cheryl, who sat stone-faced.

As with many couples, something was going on in Sam and Cheryl's interpersonal dynamics that was getting in the way of her libido. Hoping for some common and warmer ground, I had them tell their love story. Sam and Cheryl had known each other before her first husband had been killed in a car accident. Their kids competed together on the same local swim club team. In the last stages of divorcing his first wife, Sam had his eyes on Cheryl and had always enjoyed her company. Although mutual friends had warned him away while she was in mourning, he eventually couldn't resist calling her.

Cheryl, still chafing from the way the session had begun, said, "A while after my husband died and Sam's divorce was final, he called me to go to the movies—kind of out of the blue, I thought—and as they say, the rest is history. We hit it off and dated from that point forward." Then, more warmly and with a shy smile toward Sam, she continued, "I thought he had cute buns."

It was a good sign that the low-desire spouse, Cheryl, had given Sam a fairly sexual compliment. They'd known each other for an extended period of time in multiple roles and settings and still had chemistry with each other. Their relationship had a good foundation. I asked Sam about their early, good sex.

"Sex wasn't good—it was fabulous! I swear to God, I thought I'd struck gold when I found Cheryl. She had the loudest orgasms of any woman I've ever been with. Why would she want that to stop? It's crazy. She knew when she married me that sex was going to be a big deal. My first marriage lasted sixteen years and sex was a problem for us too. It wasn't the reason I left, but maybe I should have left because of it. Cheryl and her first husband did *not* have sexual problems, so I thought I was safe," he said, frustration and hurt pouring out of him. "Now I feel a little like she's tricked me."

Is Sex That Important?

"Yes, Sam, I knew sex was important to you," said Cheryl in response to Sam's complaints, "but I really didn't think you were going to be consumed by it. Sex with my first husband, Frank, was nice, but we went on with our lives afterward. It wasn't the only thing he thought about."

And indeed, as Barry McCarthy points out in *Rekindling Desire*, sex in a functioning marriage serves its purpose to enhance vitality and satisfaction. But if your spouse has low desire, then "sexuality plays an inordinately powerful role, draining positive feelings and tearing at the marital fabric." And this was exactly what was happening with Cheryl and Sam.

With some intensity, Cheryl responded, "I think Frank and I were younger and both wanted sex more frequently. Then we developed this natural pattern. Sam and I met at a different time in our lives. I'm more tired. I went back to work when Frank died, and after I've run a couple of kids around during the afternoon and made dinner, I just want to plop."

Sam wasn't willing to dismiss the problem so readily. "I run kids around too and work full-time," he insisted. Nothing had really changed in their situation in the past two years, whereas two years ago, "she couldn't get enough of me," he added. "I think that argument is bullshit. Would you tell her that lots of women work and have kids and want sex? I've come to the conclusion that she doesn't love me and wishes we hadn't married. I think about and want sex pretty much all the time. Not just anytime, anywhere, any woman. I love Cheryl and I think about her body and making love to her all the time. You can't say, 'I love you; I just don't want to have sex with you.' That doesn't even compute in my mind."

Mergers and Acquisitions

We marry because we want closeness; we want to love and be loved. Yet at the same time we desperately want to remain our own person. We want to be respected for our separate ideas, our opinions, and our plans. Connecting securely to a partner without feeling like we are losing our sense of self can take years of marriage to work out. And Sam and Cheryl were just at the beginning.

In order to freely merge in marriage without fear of being subsumed, we need to be a whole person; we have to know who we are and know what is important to us as individuals. We must feel like we have a purpose in life that fulfills us and that our partner values this as well. Having authority to make our own decisions and set separate goals without being micromanaged gives us a sense of remaining powerful. We need enough separateness to feel like we can breathe.

Another part of us wants to be intimately known, to be unique and loved by someone special. We want to share the secrets of our souls and our innermost minds. We crave passionate intimacy with our bodies. We want to be secure in our commitment to another.

When we marry, however, these two needs often get divided into the two distinct partners. One spouse becomes the "pursuer," favoring more closeness, and the other becomes a "distancer," favoring more separateness. At times, a couple might swap roles over a particular issue. For instance, a man deeply involved in his work, in his life away from his spouse and family, may want lots of sex. A woman who wants to be closer emotionally to her husband and know everything he is feeling may not be interested in bed. They change roles over sex, but the distance between them stays constant. This distance often feels unhappy to both of them.

Pursuers often use lots of words trying to generate intensity inside the marriage. The highlight of their day is talking things over with their partner. They like to direct things and like things done right. Home and family are high priorities, with building a secure nest at the top of the list. Sometimes, their wish for reassurance causes this person to begin to "overask." For instance, they may want more time together as a family but their partner seems less interested. "Family time" becomes the major topic of conversation, how it's important, where to put it on the calendar, etc. The pursuer can become preoccupied with ensuring a supply for their needs. They will deluge their partner with requests, causing their partner to back away. Once their partner backs away, they resort to an even stronger tactic—they criticize. They express the myriad of ways that their partner fails to make things better. In their anxious state, they can exaggerate conflict and become aggressive. Their anxiety is caused by feeling deprived and deep down they are afraid of being abandoned and out of control.

Distancers favor independence. They relax by doing solo activities like exercising, working on the computer, or reading the paper. They are good responders and helpers and they like to get things done, but details are often lost on them. Succinct and to the point, they talk facts and might tire easily or get annoyed if their partner talks feelings. For many reasons, they seem to find the most intensity in life outside the relationship, often devoting the best part of their day to their profession. Perhaps because they work so much, they feel the need for adventure and get frustrated with their partner's focus on security over excitement. Most of the time they will minimize conflict because they don't worry as much about the relationship and are often baffled when their partner has a litany of complaints. When they do fight, they want their good intentions to be acknowledged. In an effort to end conflict quickly, distancers will overpromise, forget, and underdeliver. Anxiety springs from feeling smothered and their deepest fear is of being controlled and absorbed by someone else.

Sexually, pursuers are initiators—even if they are the distancer outside of the bedroom. They will risk rejection over and over hoping to bring more warmth and intimacy into the relationship. Sex is the way they feel love and best express love. It is the source of intimacy. Ideas about sexual innovation are what they live for. For a sexual pursuer, excitement is the goal, as opposed to emotional pursuers, who find security the goal. In their fantasy, sex is magically complementary—their spouse wants it when, as often as, and how they want it. They ache to be desired. "Working at the sexual relationship" seems like an oxymoron. Usually generous lovers, they tune into their partner's every sign and nuance. What-ever it takes to make their partner climax is fine; their motto—the more time spent in bed the better. Their anxiety is often about sex not being enough—not frequent enough, not passionate enough. Intensity in bed is a craving. They easily forget how much effort it takes for their partner to be ready. And they can feel im-potent rage if their partner seems to withhold this aspect of the relationship—a need that cannot be met outside their monoga-mous promise.

Sexual distancers like sex. In fact, they often find it a powerful, emotional experience. But letting go and being out of control feels intimidating. Orgasm exposes their soul. Reliability and feeling safe is far more important to the sexual distancer than having an adventure—much like their emotional pursuer counterpart. Surprisingly, they will sometimes masturbate as a way to privately manage the intensity of the experience. Seduction, on the other hand, is the interpersonal elixir that makes them brave physically. Cautiously, they enjoy sex when and where they are most com-fortable with it. They like to be prepared for it and resent sex being sprung on them. Lovemaking evolves from intimacy; it's the out-come of closeness. Each sexual occasion has its own merits and isn't compared to the future or measured against the past. In their minds, sex is one avenue to express love; its frequency is never an indicator of their commitment or attraction to their partner. They easily forget how important it is to their partner. Their part-ner's intense reactions to sex—during or after, disappointment or happiness—can surprise them. At least once, they would like to satisfy their partner completely with their sexiness, technique, and pleasure. They can feel confused and overwhelmed by their partner's rage about their sex life if several other areas of their lives seem to be going well.

Neither partner is all to blame for the distance between them. It is impossible to figure out who started it, though many couples believe it is important to do so and waste hours of therapy blaming each other. In actuality, subtle movements from both sides are necessary to maintain this distance of unhappiness. The good news is that in a reasonable, healthy marriage, even one person making the committed effort to change can force the whole dynamic to shift.

We always marry our emotional-health equal, but that person often expresses the opposite end of the closeness-distance needs spectrum. The majority of women identify more with the emotional pursuer side of the continuum, though they may find themselves on the opposite position over sex. Sam was both an emotional and sexual pursuer and Cheryl was an emotional and sexual distancer.

I asked Cheryl about what had changed in the last two years. Trying to express how subtle Sam's control was, she told me about their recent move. "It's little things. I hardly even want to bring them up. But everything is under his control. He's generous about letting me redecorate but it's paid for with checks printed with his name only."

Sam explained that although he added Cheryl's name to the account, he still had two boxes of blank checks. Rather than order new checks, he'd wait until those ran out and add Cheryl's name on the next batch of checks. He didn't care how much she spent. "I have the money," he added. The specifics of their marital dynamics were beginning to show. I asked Sam to listen to how he'd said "I have the money" rather than "We have the money." And he hadn't ordered new checks with her name on them even though it would only cost a few dollars to do so. Sam had a hard time understanding how I could nitpick over such a small event and not see how generous he had been.

"Sam, we're trying to discover ways that you crowd the space between you and Cheryl. If you can control less and back away some, she will feel less of a need to distance herself from you sexually and emotionally."

Cheryl expressed over and over the ways she felt one down in her relationship with Sam. She couldn't contribute as much money because she had taken time off to raise kids. They lived in his house. His family rules predominated. His big personality took center stage at home and with friends. Cheryl felt overshadowed in their relationship. And Sam, admittedly, did feel a little jealous of the people in Cheryl's life who had come before him: Frank, his parents, who still clamored to be part of their life, and even her children. He felt diluted by all her other priorities.

Retreating into her own world of thoughts and preoccupations felt like the only way not to be overtaken with Sam's life. Like most distancers, Cheryl wasn't a good arguer. She didn't want to push back against his encroaching demands because she was afraid it would hurt his feelings.

Distancers have a responsibility to appropriately represent themselves in a conflict. Women, culturally trained to be nurturers and to put everyone's needs before their own, are challenged by early marital negotiations. They must exercise their "voice"—they have to speak up about what they want and stand up for what feels fair in their relationship. Without a fight, women often suffer silent resentment that deadens their erotic feelings. They can unconsciously use their body to express their feelings. I worried that Cheryl's sudden low libido had resulted from her passivity in her marriage and the blending of her and Sam's families. I proposed that sexual desire was in her control and it was being muted to prevent being swamped by him.

Pursuers have to take seriously the early complaints from their partner so that they don't bulldoze through conflicts and eventually push their partner even further away. Frequently, they are quick-tongued in a struggle and have to learn to give their spouse the time necessary to formulate their argument. Time-outs, even a day or so of time, might be necessary for the distancer partner, who may be slowed by the emotional intensity of the fight.

After we'd discussed this distancer/pursuer dynamic, Cheryl offered some ideas about their sexual problems. "Before, we met each other out for the evening and only had sex in hotels or when his kids were at their mother's. We didn't want to introduce our relationship to the children unless we were sure about each other. Obviously, we designated a literal 'sex space' and that was great for me. And even though he remembers it differently, we probably only had sex once a week. Now, if we've just had sex, Sam starts fuming about how we may not have another chance to do it soon enough. Sex ends with him being mad at me instead of with relaxation and fun like it used to. No matter what I do, I'm a disappointment."

Sam's anxiety about getting enough sex ruined the time he and Cheryl had together. In point of fact, they were having sex more often, sometimes twice a week. It didn't count, he argued, because she wasn't into it. Gradually, he began to see how his disappointment was pressuring her.

"It takes maturity and experience to adjust the balance when one or both partners are feeling smothered or abandoned," write Harville Hendrix and Helen Hunt in *Receiving Love*. "The partner who wants more closeness may feel that the connection is under threat and may push for more outward signs of connectedness as reassurance that the bond is still there. The partner who wants more autonomy does not necessarily want less connection; he or she simply finds it more comfortable to be connected when there is more space in which to move and breathe."

Closeness and distance may be so delicately balanced that a slight shift destabilizes your sexual adjustment. And the way the genders interpret their differences can determine how sex weighs in the balance. For instance, a woman may feel that sex is the most intimate part of herself. After sex, she is filled with thoughts and complicated emotions. Perhaps her husband expected their encounter to be physical release, playtime, and downtime. After sex, he is relaxed and at peace. He is letting go and falling asleep, but she feels wonderfully connected and wants to deepen their bond by having an in-depth, soul-searching conversation.

Orgasm during lovemaking is the ultimate merger. It's like all the molecules inside get mixed up with someone else's molecules. For a brief moment we allow ourselves to lose the boundaries of consciousness and separateness in pure sensation. In order to fully surrender to the pleasure, we must trust that afterward our molecules will come back in rightful order. Only with mature personal development can we know this to be true and lend ourselves to the experience without fear of being irreparably scrambled.

I grew up watching *Get Smart* on television. Agent Maxwell Smart walks into CONTROL and all the various doors slam behind him. The center of his operation is guarded with top security.

Marriage is the same. Intimate love requires protecting. Thus when we fall in love, we quit having sex with others, we renounce all potential partners. We take vows of commitment. We give up our own space and change our living arrangements. We sacrifice some individual time to another's interests and values. We look forward to a special, sacred relationship.

In the beginning, though, it feels like a gamble. We may hear those doors resound loudly as they slam shut behind us. We are trapped. We suffocate a little. In reality, we do give up more autonomy in this stage than in any other phase of life except when we have infant children.

This Is Me. Who Are You?

Sam and Cheryl had found a complementary partner in each other. Though they had similar family values, Cheryl was better at the emotional complexity necessary to getting along with his children and Sam brought energy to the family, energy that got things done. When all things work together for the good of both, a couple can be an unstoppable unit, each partner bringing their respective strengths to the alliance.

As time goes by, the couple gets more and more married, so to speak, with each new sharing: bodies, space, money, time, in-laws, and children. But for Sam and Cheryl, each new commingling of their lives sharpened their anxiety over their differences. Cheryl balked at the merger and Sam tried to underplay his anxiety but pushed to have things his way. Now, in every corner of their life, the differences that had originally seemed charming and winsome drove them apart.

In therapy, we worked to redistribute many aspects of the balance in this new marriage. As I had suspected, their sexual interaction was unconsciously stuck.

In order to meet her needs for autonomy, Cheryl picked a night to be alone in her new house without any interruption. Sam's insecurities temporarily increased. He believed this need of hers for private time was a symbol of her wanting to escape him. Sam's anxiety over being abandoned in small and large ways started to emerge. I comforted him by explaining that Cheryl needed alone time for herself. "Alone time isn't really 'away-from-you time'—it's away from everything and everybody," I told him. "It's time under her own direction. She'll come back to you fueled up with more reserves and be able to feel closer."

Sex can be used to meet a variety of needs, including tension release, motivation, fantasy outlet, sleep aid, conflict resolution, and comfort—all of which are normally legitimate. But in a marriage that has a fragile equilibrium over the issue of frequency, using sex to soothe a large variety of feelings rather than just expressing sexual desire can burden the lower-desire person. Some of these needs can be met with alternatives: exercise for tension relief, regular routines around sleep times, or masturbation for immediate sexual gratification. Sex to Sam spelled reassurance. But he needed to grow in his ability to comfort himself when Cheryl was away, whether she was unavailable by actual absence or by being preoccupied. He needed to hold his anxiety in check so that it stopped wrinkling the sheets.

Sam's panting availability made him overly familiar to Cheryl and left her feeling crowded. As sex therapist Esther Perel in *Mating in Captivity* poetically expresses it: "Love enjoys knowing everything about you: desire needs mystery . . . too often as couples settle into the comforts of love, they cease to fan the flame of desire. They forget that fire needs air."

I suggested that Cheryl initiate sex once a week when she was ready for it and when the moment was best for her. Even though one part of her had shut off her libido in frustration, another part of her was attracted to all of Sam's energy. She needed to take some action that would prove to Sam that she wanted the marriage to be sexual. Since they could afford to rent a hotel room and it seemed like a fabulous escape from their children, I asked her why she had given up the idea. She admitted that she thought it might seem tawdry to sneak away from her responsibilities. We had to rework her sense of entitlement to play. Sexually, she began to flirt with Sam to feed his wish to be desired so his hunger didn't grow to such proportions that he would invade her. She got in touch with things she found erotic. She'd dance with him in their kitchen. She watched romantic movies on her nights off. And she booked an adults-only away weekend once a quarter. She needed to come forward as much as he needed to back up.

I further urged her to say what bothered her rather than disappearing into the "good wife" role. Ironically, Sam calmed down and felt safe whenever she directly asked for what she wanted rather than trying harder to just get along.

As we delved more deeply into Cheryl's previous marriage, it turned out that it wasn't totally satisfying after all. Flaws that Frank's premature death had led her to gloss over came to light. While it had been happy, they had never really thought to change things, even for the better—neither spouse had been as interested in examination as Sam. She began to appreciate how Sam had a more intense desire to know her mind as well as her body than Frank had had. We talked about how this drew Cheryl into the romance with Sam. While she and Frank had had an easy companionship, Sam shared more of himself and offered more emotional intimacy than would have ever been possible in her previous marriage.

The Between Place

The ability to contain your own worries and anxieties is coined by David Schnarch, Ph.D., author of *Passionate Marriage*, as "holding onto yourself." Our first instinctual reactions when feeling uncomfortable about how close or distant our spouse is can be to start pestering, or to start running. Our anxiety has us frantically seeking our own interests without considering the feelings and interests of our mate and ironically enforcing a pattern that leaves us unhappy. When we call a halt to our own unconscious reaction, we can then think more clearly, act more directly, and find a better balance—between our self-interest and our concern for our partner.

Despite the frustration of feeling like nothing satisfies their partner, an emotional distancer needs to make small changes in response to their partner's requests. For instance, initiating a conversation about the events of the day, putting the phone down during dinner, planning a date, managing the children all day on a Saturday, and paying attention to details. For sexual distancers, picking a time in their own mind to make love once a week and planning a creative sexual escapade will make a sexual pursuer happy.

Even if it seems your partner is starving you purposely, a pursuer must hold on to themselves so that their partner feels safe enough to come closer. Keeping critical words to themselves is the number one thing a pursuer can do to change the relationship for the better. They need to accept imperfect change and stop keeping score. Getting what they want sometimes makes pursuers nervous; they must stop dithering over whether their partner's transformation is authentic or permanent. Finding other hobbies, interests, and friendships that nurture them will alleviate the temporary feelings of emptiness. Sexual pursuers should compliment every lovemaking experience rather than finding ways to improve it.

It's hard to change once we've become suspicious that our partner might ignore or trample our desires if we meet their needs. Believing that our partner is selfish is the hallmark of the power struggle in marriage. Balancing our needs as a couple has to come from the desire to love. Sex, particularly, doesn't bear concession well. If a person feels that they have extracted something grudgingly from the other, the gift doesn't count. We defend by saying, "But I gave you what you want!" and we mask our surprise that our partner could see through our offering to our heart's resentment. When negotiating these issues of connection and autonomy, pursuit and distance, we cannot resort to a trade. The bargain of "I'll have sex with you twice a week if you take me on a date night and help more around the house" is rejected by our souls. We want someone who is delighted to spend time with us and who glories in our body and, in turn, someone we're delighted to be with. Honoring the relationship means that there is a place between us that is beyond compromise. We work toward true understanding rather than quid pro quo. We commit to changing ourselves regardless of our partner's response, without waiting for reciprocity. It's a place that we risk "going first" for, not waiting for evidence of change. We value the relationship as being greater than the sum of its parts. Though we didn't know it would cost us so much, we change for love's sake. And even if the relationship doesn't work out, our changes—for instance, a woman investing in her own eroticism—often make our own lives better and more complete.

Help Yourself

1. Are you a sexual pursuer (initiates, craves closeness, criticizes) or a sexual distancer (responds, needs space, withdraws)? Does the dynamic change for emotional closeness between you and your partner?

2. For sexual pursuers, name three things your lover is good at in bed.

3. For sexual distancers, describe a turndown to a sexual overture that would reassure your partner of your desire for them.

4. Do you feel an imbalance in your relationship in areas other than sex? Discuss any way you feel sex might be speaking for other issues that need more direct negotiation.

5. List two ways your partner has asked you to change. What are the costs and benefits involved in this change?

CHAPTER THREE

The Big, Elusive O: Getting to Orgasm

Sarah—brunette, blue-eyed, slight of frame, and twenty-seven years old—was wearing a simple A-line skirt, sweater, and kitten heels when she came to see me. In response to a question about libido, her insightful gynecologist had asked her, after a thorough physical exam, "Do you have orgasms?" Married four years, Sarah had never had one. Not by herself, not with a partner. Women need orgasms to have libido.

For men, sexual activity—barring dysfunction—results in orgasm. When I begin treatment with a couple, I help the man gain perspective by asking how many times a week, how many weeks, and for how many years would he want to have sex if he were allowed only to thrust but never to climax? The question is ludicrous, but the answer sheds light on the joint problem.

Men shouldn't feel guilty about the ease and regularity of their orgasms. Wonderfully, the sexual reliability of their genital response feeds desire and pleasure. And most men want their partners to reach orgasm too. In fact, men often say witnessing a woman surrendering to climax is the sexiest part of lovemaking. Her turn-on is his biggest turn-on. Seeing excitement reflected multiplies the thrill.

Unfortunately, men don't always have enough knowledge to help their partners reach the Big O. Nor should they assume all responsibility. Locker-room exchanges don't typically include how to touch a woman's clitoris. They wouldn't have heard about it from their fathers during the infamous sex talk at thirteen. Porn often shows endless penetration shots that lead both men and women to reach false conclusions about what truly brings women to climax. Even more sadly, some men have erroneously come to believe that women don't need orgasms.

Frustration occurs, then, on both sides. Women aren't having orgasms and men are lost about how to help. If a woman doesn't have sufficient knowledge of her body to know or communicate what she needs, she's going to have a hard time reaching climax. Lack of orgasm can make a woman ambivalent about sex. Although she dreads disappointing her lover, he senses her lukewarm response. She wonders what all the fuss is about. Yet many women expect themselves to want sex under exactly such circumstances, and do have repeated sex, year after year, most weeks, sometimes several times a week, without a climax.

Certainly, orgasm is not all we need. An orgasmic woman can describe more complex needs met by sex: emotional connection, intimacy, relatedness, even spiritual oneness. Occasionally, she may want to experience the closeness of a sexual exchange without coming herself, which is her prerogative. But without climaxing as the norm? Sex becomes a dull prospect. Libido dies.

All in Good Time

Even women who have previously had orgasms while dating may find, once married, that they are no longer able to come. Nine times out of ten, the halt signifies not enough time for pleasure, touch, and caresses. Women who say they are not orgasmic often mean they can have one by themselves but not with a partner. Comparing themselves to their male partner, women think there is something wrong with themselves because it takes so long for them to climax. But men and women are radically different in their response times.

Misconceptions about how women orgasm can also lead to technique failures that limit the frequency of their climaxes. Nearly every movie shows women reaching orgasm through sexual intercourse alone in a minute's clip. In reality, only about 15 to 20 percent of women reach orgasm through penile-vaginal thrusting. Even then, much of the pleasure comes from the pressing, tapping, tugging, and movement that intercourse generates for her clitoris.

Innumerable women have said to me, almost as though they're apologizing for a personal flaw, "I can orgasm, but only with foreplay. I can't do it with sex." It's as if these women think an orgasm with direct clitoral stimulation is second rate. It's not! It's the way most women come. It's why we have a clitoris!

If couples believe intercourse itself is the ultimate—and only rightful—expression of lovemaking, several misconceptions about sex automatically follow. Pleasuring is called foreplay because it's thought of as getting ready for "the real thing." Making out has to progress to be meaningful to such couples. Sensual play can seem frustrating if it's simply a prelude to the main act. Any erotic behavior other than intercourse is seen as diminishing. Individual lovemaking sessions may end when intercourse is over whether she is satisfied or not. "Everything but" doesn't count. But without plenty of flexibility and latitude, sexual encounters are cut off too soon, or are simply avoided on days when intercourse might be deemed impossible or undesirable. This takes a lot of the playfulness out of a couple's sex life.

Women are not the only ones hurt by these erroneous assumptions. Focusing on intercourse may put pressure on a male who is struggling with early ejaculation. He feels pressure to last longer inside her vagina, and the more pressure he feels, the more anxious he becomes and the faster he climaxes. Later in life, ordinary incidents of erectile dysfunction are met with great dismay because the invariable formula prescribing that all touches lead to intercourse is suddenly changed.

When the Big O Is a Total Stranger

Sarah admitted that she had no one else with whom to discuss her concern. Simply put, she didn't have orgasms. Even without climaxing, Sarah still appreciated the warmth she and her husband, Terry, felt as a couple after intercourse, but that didn't reassure Terry. He felt responsible for making it happen for his wife. Later he admitted that he had wondered if he was inadequate in terms of size and had felt deep shame. He'd become so discouraged that he'd almost stopped initiating altogether.

"Sex happens when he's desperate," explained Sarah, "mainly just quickies now. He says he feels bad even bothering me with it.

You probably think I'm stupid for having waited four years to do anything about this."

I didn't think she was stupid; I thought she needed fast, practical help. Anorgasmia—inability to orgasm—usually has an easy fix. Sarah told me that they tried manual stimulation and oral sex, but neither had brought about the desired result. I asked how long foreplay usually lasted. Sarah's reply added valuable information we could work with.

"When we were dating we didn't have sex because of our beliefs," she began. "So all we did was touch and fool around and I was definitely turned on. I seriously looked forward to intercourse. I would almost reach some sort of cliff's edge back then, though never quite tip over.

"Then, from our wedding night forward, the whole focus changed to intercourse. It hurt initially, and later it didn't feel particularly . . . well, particularly anything. I felt tense the whole honeymoon. Never really relaxed then, I suppose. We were both tremendously disappointed. But I still wanted to be with Terry. I love him and could see how much pleasure he got from the whole thing. I hoped that I would start to climax too, after a while.

"Except it all went downhill from there. Now I would say foreplay lasts about five minutes."

They'd utterly given up all the lovely, arousing caresses of their premarital experience. That explained a lot about what went wrong. I asked if "five minutes" meant total time spent on trying to get her aroused or directly on her genitals after she already felt aroused.

"Total." Gulp.

I asked her to give me the most detailed scenario that she felt comfortable conveying.

"Terry usually rolls over in bed," she said, "and starts rubbing me between my legs." With no buildup, he would immediately touch her vulva. Did that feel good?

"No, I feel nothing. Once he works his way between my labia, it even feels a little painful."

Men Are Different

When a woman is touched intimately while she's not yet aroused, she frequently feels very little or even feels irritated. If she's dry, which would be normal before arousal, touch can feel too sensitive or raw. And it can feel invasive to have sex initiated that way. A man, however, could be touched in a flaccid state and be quickly excited. In fact, I think most husbands would feel they'd won the lottery if their wives just grabbed their penis to start a sexual encounter. That's why Terry used such a direct approach with Sarah—it's what he'd want. Once men realize that their wife's clitoris needs to be stimulated, they get down to business.

The problem is that most women don't turn on that way. They need to be somewhat aroused before they like their genitals touched. Seductive undressing, long, slow body caressing, skin on skin, sexy talking, and lusty kissing—all these help build appetite. Remember that high school sense of urgency? And long after graduation, a woman is ignited by the man with an insatiable craving for her. "Women want to be thrown up against a wall but not truly endangered. Women want a caveman and caring," postulates Marta Meana, researcher and professor of psychology at University of Nevada, Las Vegas. While she apologized for the anti-feminist sounding idea, Meana believes that a woman's desire gets sparked by being the object of her partner's excitement. Women want sexual energy from a focused man.[1]

After I explained how female arousal works, Sarah let out a sigh of relief. She had been holding her breath, and now she exhaled. "Really? I guess I thought I was just broken. When he starts touching me, I kind of clam up. Then he'll roll back to his side of the bed, like I'm a dead fish. I feel so guilty."

His let-down didn't inspire arousal in her. My heart went out to Sarah. She'd held to her standards before marriage, and she expected that she would automatically be rewarded with great sex after the wedding. Alas, while her ethics remained intact, her dreams of easy, effortless lovemaking had been shattered.

Some people wait until the wedding to have sex because of their faith or cultural commitments. I see many Indian clients in arranged marriages that face starting their marriage as strangers, both with a complete lack of sexual education and mounting parental pressure for grandchildren in unions that have not been consummated at all. Often these women are extremely anxious about intercourse because of cultural inhibitions about talking about sex.

The ideal of having only one partner can mean both bride and groom are learners. Neither of them has any prior experience for comparison. The sexual adjustment period is going to extend far beyond the honeymoon. These couples should be advised that sexual harmony will take a lot longer to achieve than one wedding night.

Education Pays

Sex takes effort and attention—work (though a delicious kind, I assure you), if you will—whenever it starts. Waiting until marriage to have sex should not mean a delay in education and communication. Couples can prepare by reading sexual instruction books, completing workbooks, taking classes, and by talking about sex with each other. Consulting a therapist with a sexual specialization can help equip both partners with realistic expectations. They should explicitly tell each other their hopes and dreams about the wedding night. If the couple has turned off their sexual desire in order to have a long, chaste engagement, they cannot expect to turn sexual feelings instantly back on at the altar. Religious couples, especially those who might have progressed further sexually while dating than their standards permitted, need to work through their guilt in order to forgive themselves and enter the intimate arena of marriage freely. Many times the root of low desire in these faith-filled couples comes from self-punishment over unprocessed guilt.

Some women also worry that intercourse will be painful, and indeed, fear of pain is a desire killer. Virgins can prepare themselves and markedly reduce any pain with first intercourse. First have a thorough exam by a gynecologist to ensure that penetration will not be obstructed by a hymen that is too tough or blocking the entrance of the vagina. Then, by following a prescribed series of progressively deeper and wider manual stretching of your vaginal tissue, you will minimize the pain of the pending intercourse. Begin in the shower by inserting one finger slowly and gently into the opening of your vagina. Push your finger toward the perineum (the space between your vagina and anus) to stretch the vaginal vestibule (entrance). Women who follow a complete course of stretching experience no or very little pain on first intercourse. Women's health physical therapists are practitioners who specialize in the reduction of all kinds of pelvic and genital pain and are experts in teaching these exercises.

Orgasm for a woman is complicated; it requires self-knowledge, time, and technique. I asked Sarah to tell me what used to happen when she felt herself becoming highly excited. She used to get close, she replied. But then at a certain point, her legs would snap shut. And then it nearly hurt to be touched.

Indeed, she probably was quite close to climaxing. Near the point of orgasm, women often describe a threshold where the pleasure is so intense that it can be almost unbearable. Rather than trying to keep her legs open when they "seemed to have a will of their own," as she put it, I suggested she let her legs do what they wanted since stimulation could still continue. First we'd isolate the various issues, I explained to her, and then we'd work on that particular concern later.

Surprised, Sarah asked, "But he won't be able to be inside, then? I want to be able to orgasm the real way. And I've heard that orgasms are best when he's inside."

Not necessarily.

Inside, Outside, Upside Down

Many women report that clitoral stimulation produces the best orgasm. And as we've already discussed, intercourse alone may or may not produce an orgasm. Certainly, there can be a different feeling when an orgasm happens with vaginal penetration, but intensity is subjective for each woman and even from orgasm to orgasm in the same woman.

For the record, here's how to aim for the biggest orgasm: have a huge amount of clitoral stimulation with varying amounts of pressure, some of it even teasing, hold right on the edge of orgasm, and go over the cliff only when you can't stand the tension a second longer.

A man may like his testicles gently handled and touched for stimulation, but he definitely wants his penis to be touched too! Similarly, a woman's vagina feels good when penetrated but her clitoris is even more responsive. In a smaller area, the glans of the clitoris—the pealike bulb covered with a tissue hood on the tip—has an even more highly concentrated number of nerve endings than the head of the penis. The tip of the clitoris has enormous potential for exquisite sensation, both good and bad. It is far too delicate ever to be touched dry.

Actually, the visible part of the clitoris is like the floating tip of an iceberg. The clitoral legs extend deep into the pelvic area like a wishbone structure and respond to the pressure of touch as well. Obviously, the visible part of the clitoris is the most straightforward path to these nerves. Vaginal penetration can stimulate the deep legs of the clitoris from underneath. Certainly, the vagina has sexual pleasure nerves too, mostly at the outer third closest to the opening. She has has the highly sensitive G-spot in the vagina located on the roof beneath her urethra, and that can feel very delightful when stimulated by her partner's penis or fingers. The G-spot is actually a spongy part of the clitoral structure. Deeper areas are gratified when stretched and stimulated via intercourse. But the vagina is not an inside-out penis like many men have imagined.

"I think Terry would feel so left out if he's not inside me," worried Sarah. She would not be dissuaded from the goal of intercourse-induced orgasm. In her mind, there was a right way for sex to take place. Often, a woman has a particular goal, even though, over time, the more sexual flexibility a couple has, the more they are able to sustain loving, erotic connection through the slings and arrows that life shoots their way. Fluidity in lovemaking, in all its forms, is sex insurance.

Sarah believed that the ultimate sexual experience was simultaneous orgasm. While it may be glorious when simultaneous orgasm happens, men and women move differently when they climax, which can be a distraction from the ecstasy of what each is feeling. In an early sexual relationship, the satisfaction and closeness of both lovers is a better immediate goal than having it all happen simultaneously. Although I could coach Sarah on the positions most likely to give her a "hands-off" orgasm eventually, her past experience with Terry already proved this would be an unlikely outcome.

Penetration-only orgasms are likely to happen in two positions:

1. Woman on her back (on a relatively hard surface like carpet, as a bed changes the angle of her hips) with her legs wrapped around the man's elbows. For the young and gymnastically adventurous, she can hook knees around his shoulders. This angle tips her pelvis and hopefully allows maximum friction on her G-spot by his penis. She could also place pillows under her hips to change their elevation.

2. Woman on top leaning forward about forty-five degrees. She finds the best connective angle internally and can ad-

just so that her clitoris receives lots of contact with his pelvis. If simultaneous orgasm is the goal, then she can reach down and touch herself or ask him to also touch her clitoris in any position. Vibrators too are useful for intense clitoral stimulation during intercourse so that the two can orgasm closer to the same time.

To understand what Sarah's ideal of mutual climax actually meant, I asked her to imagine lovemaking with Terry, both of them reaching the pinnacle at once, and to describe her feelings.

"I think I would feel fulfilled. Not just physically, but emotionally and maybe spiritually, to be so connected and so absorbed all at once. I always imagined something like that for my wedding night and, of course, we're well past that. I guess it would mean we were married."

She saw two souls merging. She hungered for the togetherness that sexual intercourse and simultaneous orgasm would represent. I wondered if she felt left out, then, since Terry had been climaxing for the last four years without her, and asked her as much.

"Mmm, maybe I do. It seems the whole world knows something I don't." She was clearly disappointed to have waited for this special experience, only to have it not happen.

"Maybe I just imagined it would be something that isn't possible," she confided. "I thought sex would be more 'fade-to-black' and less sweat and muscle. I didn't expect all this nitty-gritty technique work. Nothing about it feels natural or ladylike. I feel humiliated to confess this, but we knew so little about what we were doing, we even came apart when we first had intercourse. I was afraid he'd hurt himself trying to get back in the right place."

I couldn't help smiling as I replied, "Coming apart is about the most natural and common experience of new lovers! All couples have to find their rhythm and stride."

She was right too about the logistics of sexuality. On the surface, sex is limbs splayed, one messy, sweaty, body-fluidy commingling. More earthy than heavenly. And more woman than lady.

Down Here on Earth

Sarah resisted the notion of focusing on herself and her body to learn how to orgasm: "I've been taught that masturbation is withholding and selfish." I disagreed, though not openly, and know that most women discover orgasm for themselves through masturbation. Sarah was particularly anxious about selfishness because she saw it as the opposite of love. She'd also been taught that sex is about serving the other, not about the mutual pleasure that reinforces love.

Is it selfish, as Sarah suspected, for a woman to focus on herself? Hardly. Women tend to worry about sins of omission, as feminist Carol Gilligan says, "of not helping others when you could."[2] Female moral maturity means considering it right to treat herself an equal to others in the desire to help and not hurt people. Orgasm for a woman requires times of self-absorption. Men and women both must revel in selfish separateness during sexual ecstasy right at the moment of deep union—a moment of separateness amid attachment.[3] Later Sarah could focus on other aspects of the sex act, like what pleased Terry, how to initiate, or specific techniques. Without orgasm, though, her libido would suffer over the long haul. Then her husband would suffer too. Sarah needed this external motivation to move her past her anxious fears. Good sex needs us to be concerned about our own pleasure.

In another session, Terry came with Sarah to learn how he could improve in technique. They'd already made some big changes by setting aside Saturday nights for dinner out and lovemaking. Sarah explained to Terry how much foreplay most women need, and he realized he had been remiss. "I used to think learning about sex from books was like learning to ride a bike from reading!" he admitted, but now he bought some books on sex and dove into them.

"My only other relationship lasted all of two months," he explained, "and I don't know if that girl climaxed or not. I was way too guilty and immature to ever talk about that with her. I think some of my turning away from Sarah after an unsuccessful lovemaking session was my own disgust at my inadequacy as a lover. I was raised like Sarah, and we never talked about sex at home. My older sister got pregnant in high school, and my parents felt like it ruined their standing in the church. They still seem to hang their heads in shame at Christmas Eve services that we all attend when we go home for the holidays. They love their grandson to pieces and didn't make my sister marry his father, but the whole incident made a serious impression on me as a teenager. I made sure I used a condom during my one fling."

In essence, as much as Terry felt responsible, he didn't have much experience either. Even sexually "experienced" men enter therapy only to learn that they have no specific knowledge about how a woman orgasms. Experience doesn't equate to expertise.

I also assured Terry that penis size has less to do with internal orgasms than the angles of the two body parts together. Any time a couple tells me that the husband has good technique, I ask how he learned his lessons. Invariably, the answer is that a previous lover or his wife gave him point-by-point, lights-on instructions about how she liked to be touched. Female bodies are so complex, it takes a lot of relaxed exploration to become an expert lover.

Small Changes = Big Impact

Sarah and Terry started to make progress. They used their dinnertime to flirt and reflect on their relationship away from the week's worries. After spending their youth trying not to be turned on or turn anyone else on, they shyly started using sexual innuendos with each other. They experimented with texting sexy messages. On the way home from their dinner date, Terry would park along a skyline or in a wooded area and they would touch and make out like they did when they were dating. He told me that he looked forward to scouting out a new place each week, as a kind of secret mission. I explained how women in long-term relationships responded to sexual drive targeted at them from their beloved. Letting go of his guilt and prior disappointment, Terry started to get in touch with his inner caveman and told and showed Sarah how much she turned him on.

He also learned to attend to small clues about Sarah's arousal progression. With information gleaned from books and our sessions, he started understanding her. He liked it when she shut her eyes because he knew she was getting excited. When he touched her genitals, he would switch his touch from the glans of her clitoris to the sides of her clitoris if she started to breathe a little heavier in order to slow it down for her. They both were instructed to ignore her legs closing and to continue touching unless Sarah gave the signal that she couldn't take any more. When she reached a certain pain-pleasure threshold, he found he could still touch her clitoris with his tongue: a soft, wet sensation that she welcomed.

"I tell her to take her time," he relayed with a grin. And once Sarah stopped trying to keep her legs from automatically closing during sex, she was able to identify what she was thinking about when it did happen.

"I feel like I'm going to pee. Every fiber in me just throws on the brakes. When Terry keeps stimulating me, it feels good, but I am overwhelmed with 'bad-girl' vibes. I sometimes just have to shove him away from me."

Sarah was afraid she'd wet the bed. What would be so terrible about that? I asked.

"It'd be the worst, most shameful thing I can imagine," she blurted. "Wow! Did I just say that?" Now she heard the truth of her fears for the first time.

Sometimes early toilet training that is too rigid can create sexual problems. Sarah noted that her mother bragged to this day that Sarah had been potty-trained in one day and never had an accident. As an exercise, I asked her to learn to either urinate in the shower or when walking in the woods.

"You're crazy." She laughed. "No good southern girl pees in the shower. And the woods? I couldn't even dream about it!" We all laughed. There is a similarity between approaching orgasm and the urgency to go to the bathroom, but they're not the same thing, no matter what your mind thinks, I reassured her. Then we tried to find something that would relax her so that her mind would stop being anxious.

"Maybe if I put down a rubber waterproof mat and lots of towels?" If that helped alleviate worry, fine.

A Vibrator as a Helping Hand

A good way to cut down on anxiety about your body's reactions is to bring yourself to orgasm without your partner present. Self-stimulation provides a perfect biofeedback loop to learn touches that increase arousal. Because some expressions of faith forbid masturbation, and because Sarah had not been open to the idea earlier in treatment, even after weeks of therapy, I asked gently here.

She surprised me by interrupting to ask about the use of vibrators. I suggested a massager that was available online, one not specifically promoted as a vibrator. It has a phallic shape, though it is not used inside the vagina, and the more powerful frequency of its vibrations works better for many women than the buzz of some vibrators sold as sex toys. Vibrators may conjure racy images of large silicone dildos bought in stores with pierced-tongue clerks by women brave enough to wear stilettos and leopard print. They're items we'd want our girlfriends to come over and destroy should we die accidentally.

Actually, nearly 60 percent of American women own vibrators. Sexuality expert Laura Berman advocated "vibrators for every woman!" during an *Oprah* episode focused on women's remarkable response potential. Some vibrators are graphically phallic-shaped with every bell and whistle, and others are so benign, pastel, and non-sexually-shaped that your children might think them a kitchen utensil. As shy as many low-libido women often are, vibrators can be ordered online and arrive in brown paper packages so the neighbors would never guess.

A vibrator can quickly help a woman know what an orgasm feels like and shorten the process of self-education. By learning to have an orgasm at your own hands, you can pick up techniques you can easily teach to your partner. And there's no need to worry about a vibrator creating sexual dependency. It's unlikely because nothing feels quite so wonderful as a gentle lover's touch.

Try these strategies for using a vibrator to help your love life:

- If it's your first time experimenting with a vibrator, begin first through a quilt or blankets. Then apply the vibrator progressively closer to the skin on top of your clitoris as you become more aroused.

- If you struggle with the whole getting-started process when you're with your mate, use the vibrator on yourself, up to but short of orgasm. Since inhibition drops naturally with high arousal, turn yourself on and then invite your husband to bed.

- Help yourself reach high arousal quickly at the beginning of a lovemaking session by using a vibrator on yourself or having your mate use one on you, with you calling the shots.

- Vibrators can complement quickies so that you too can have an orgasm.

- Use a vibrator to help resolve differences in your and your husband's expectations over frequency. Quickies become more fun and more, so to speak, participatory for you.

It Works!

Sarah and Terry arrived smiling at my office for their next visit a month later.

"I had an orgasm!" said Sarah, newfound confidence in her voice. "It happened so fast, I didn't know what hit me. Terry was shocked."

"She didn't pee either," interjected Terry. "We've basically been experimenting since."

"He's trying to tell you we had one together!" said Sarah, with what I would almost call a flirty smirk. "I was on top and leaned forward a little bit. He got so excited by me and the vibrations that he couldn't stop himself. I couldn't stop myself either."

"That's what you wanted, right? How did it feel?"

"It was nice."

"Just nice?"

With a small smile, Sarah continued: "Perhaps the heavens didn't open the way I thought they might, but this whole process is really what's made me feel married. Of course, I'm thrilled that we made it happen together at least once. What matters to me now is that we are having exciting sex. It's the sex I imagined when we were dating."

Her legs still snap together at times, but they ignore it and go on. "I usually orgasm first and then Terry enters me," Sarah said happily.

Lack of orgasm is one of the easiest sexual problems to resolve. While some women believe they may be the one unique person in the universe who can't have one, only the rare circumstances of severe trauma, spinal-cord injury, or extreme hormonal disruption would truly bar someone from the experience. And even then there have been breakthroughs that allow some to experience rerouted climaxes. Nearly every woman who *walks* through my office can have an orgasm even if she hasn't.

While Sarah was most comfortable using a vibrator, a woman using her hands to bring herself to orgasm has the advantage of incorporating her genitals more intimately into her body image.

Here is the same progression I suggested to Sarah for further exploring and getting to know her own body:

- If you've never washed your genitals with bare hands while bathing, you might try this first.

- Ensure you have some private time when you will not be interrupted, and lie down comfortably in your own bed. Allow your mind to think sexy thoughts. Without mental engagement, all the touching in the world will not ignite the body.

- Use mirrors to examine the structure of your genitals. Find a drawing of the inner vulva and identify each area on yourself. You will soon know where the shaft and glans of your clitoris are and will be able to confidently put your fingers in your vagina.

- Touch your breasts and genitals in general cupping ways to see if this arouses any sensation.

- Try smoothing oil over your whole body, including your stomach, breasts, vulva, and inner thighs, with broad smooth motions.

- Practice deep breathing and audible moaning and sighing in order to free your responsiveness.

- When you're ready, begin to stimulate your labia and clitoris. Start with even circular touches and varying pressures. Always use a lubricant. A personal silicone-based type will not be absorbed into the skin and will grant continuous glide.

First and foremost, a woman has to learn her own body for desire to even begin. Partners can help by setting aside time for long sessions of touch designed only to pleasure her—not to necessarily end in orgasm or intercourse. Without the pressure of trying to reach orgasm, a woman can relax and enjoy the touch as long as it remains pleasurable. Have the stimulation last thirty to forty-five minutes or longer, switching technique if the touch is unpleasant. Once orgasm occurs, it becomes more easily repeatable and a higher likelihood of orgasm will help restore libido.

Help Yourself

1. When and how did you learn to orgasm?

2. Have you had more difficulty at certain times? How about with your current partner?

3. Do you climax during intercourse? If not, is that a concern of yours? Of your partner's?

4. Are you satisfied with your mate's sexual technique? Are you always able to let him know how you feel or would like to feel? Use a number rating system from one to five to tell him what touch feels good.

5. Have you found ways to integrate a vibrator into your sexual repertoire?

6. Do you feel your cultural or family background has made your sexual adjustment more challenging? Describe your religious beliefs and how they impact your sexuality.

7. Discuss with your lover three favorite touches or rhythms that reliably arouse you.

CHAPTER FOUR

Kiss What?! Conflicts over Specific Acts

S exual negotiations over *what* to do in bed are often difficult in early marriage. Anxiety and conflict over the preferences of their partner can dampen the desire of many women. Being considered a good lover is important to everyone's sexual self-esteem, and when their partner criticizes or is continuously disappointed in bed, some women give up.

Any number of specific acts can be reason enough to argue about and bring a halt to early sexual relations. Arguments over giving and receiving oral sex seem to snag many couples into a stalemate that stops their enjoyment, so I've chosen this topic to focus on as an example of sexual negotiations.

Women who cannot reach orgasm through means other than cunnilingus sometimes become loath to receive it either because they feel dirty—literally or figuratively—or they know that they must reciprocate and they dislike performing fellatio. Feeling squeamish over giving oral sex leaves them hopeless about being a pleasing partner. When exquisite pleasure goes missing in a relationship for any reason, the couple's erotic bond may become frayed.

Jeff and Hannah, college sweethearts now in their late twenties, recently moved from Michigan to the South seeking milder winters and more affordable homes. They both struck me as pleasant, humorous, and smart. They were in therapy with me for a few weeks when Jeff's complaint settled on two issues: Hannah's unwillingness to perform oral sex and the couple's low sexual frequency.

"I'm sure this whole process takes time, but we've been coming for weeks, and we don't have sex any more often than we did before," began Jeff.

Asked how often they typically have sex, Hannah estimated "once a week." As often happens, a low-libido partner overestimates and a high-libido partner underestimates the answer to this question.

"No," Jeff complained. "I don't think we'd be here if it were that often. Last weekend, your folks were visiting and the weekend before you had your period. Hannah, it's been three weeks since we've had sex."

"True, but once, in between, I gave you a hand job."

"Hon, you were half asleep and I had to finish myself, if you recall. And you never do blow jobs anymore. I don't get that. You gave them all the time when we were dating."

But When We Dated, You . . .

Striving to use the good listening skills we had worked on, Hannah took a deep breath and reflected aloud: "You're upset that we don't have sex more often and that I don't give you oral sex as often as in college.".

She did an impressive job of summarizing her husband's feelings. Indeed, some of Jeff's upset dissipated, and he became willing to reveal more of his root fear.

"Yeah. I go down on you! Why don't you do it to me? I worry that you're not attracted to me anymore."

"But I *am* attracted to you, and I like it when you give me oral sex. You know that's the only way I climax."

Did you notice how Jeff used modern slang while Hannah stayed with more proper sexual language? They hadn't found a common erotic language yet. For now, I used words according to Hannah's preference in order to press ahead on her resistance to oral sex.

"Do you not like to give oral sex, Hannah?"

"No." She sighed. "I don't really." I asked her what she didn't like about it.

"What is there to like?" she replied. "I don't want you to take this the wrong way, Jeff, because it's not you. In fact, I think your body is beautiful. I just don't really want to do that." Slumping and looking back at me, she added, "And even when we have sex, he seems disappointed, so I just feel like quitting sex."

Jeff slouched on the couch too. To many men, a generous lover gives oral sex. A woman who desires a man sort of worships his penis. Even when men don't climax easily with oral sex, it remains an important part of lovemaking for them. Oral sex feels exquisite to both genders, barring preconceived feelings that might interrupt their sensations.

Looking depressed, Jeff started to say something, but I interrupted to ask Hannah to be more specific.

Finally, she answered flatly and honestly, "I don't like the smell or the taste. One time, Jeff came in my mouth and I thought that was totally disgusting. And it takes so long . . . sometimes it takes twenty minutes and my jaw gets sore. I have this really sensitive gag reflex, so I find myself choking all the time. Plus, I have images of some skanky girls we've seen on porn films spitting on their partners' penises or drooling on them. I just think it's all so base."

Jeff, hurt, responded bitterly, "I figured she didn't like giving blow jobs. I'd ask her but she was never straightforward with me." Setting his jaw and making his face go blank, he turned to Hannah and said, "I never came in your mouth."

"You did. It was in college, in my dorm room, during one of the first times I did it to you." Hannah's pitch was higher.

Apparently, she remembered tasting semen that one time and not liking it. Jeff was angry and hurt because he knew deep down that she had been deflecting his questions about liking oral sex. Though tact is paramount during discussions like these, Hannah had never talked plainly about her feelings. It's impossible to work on a problem if it's not clear what the problem is.

"I feel terrible," she said. "I always knew he wanted oral sex, and I just thought I'd be able to work myself up for it again. Obviously, that hasn't happened and now he feels rejected even more."

"I feel horrible too," seconded Jeff. "What does she mean she doesn't like my smell or taste? That's ridiculous. Sex has smells and tastes—it's what makes it sex. I can't imagine a future life without oral sex. It'd be like hugging and no kissing. This is so depressing. I wish we'd never started counseling."

Risking All

Now Jeff took the risk of confronting Hannah. "Are you saying you won't ever want to give a blow job at all? Because if you are, I'm going to have to rethink being together."

Alarmed, Hannah asked, "Seriously, Jeff? You'd throw everything we have away because I won't give you oral sex? I guess I could try again, but I'm not going to be able to try it if I feel like it's a test about whether you'll stay with me or not. I'm already super anxious about the whole thing."

There would likely be intermediate steps before this couple would show up in divorce court, but clearly, this was an opportunity for change. I got their attention, and they both looked toward me with some relief.

Every couple has to grapple with specifics. Now out in the open, her avoidance of direct negotiation and his disappointment made them both liable to withdraw from the relationship.

Loving our partner can mean stretching through uncomfortable moments to grow sexually so that we can incorporate a wider range of acts. Hannah knew how important oral sex was to her because it was the only way she came. She was willing to try to change, but she wanted an equal commitment from Jeff to give up his expectations if her efforts were unsuccessful and his needs not fully met.

It is frightening to think that the lack of one sexual act could mean the end of a relationship. It's possible that Hannah wouldn't be able to overcome her current distaste for giving oral sex. But for many men, this does feel like a core rejection. Oral sex feels like meat and potatoes to most men, not some exotic dessert to be had only on rare occasions. Prenegotiated guarantees just aren't possible.

With oral sex, there are lots of techniques to help resolve the various reasons for resistance. Hannah decided she was open to trying, making it clear that she wanted Jeff to be happy. While she could hardly fathom that he would want out of the relationship over this, she began to recognize how important it was to him. Adjustments can't begin until we hear the depth of our partner's feelings. If we feel reluctant about performing a specific erotic act, we won't have the motivation to change unless we fully understand what our partner feels.

Rallying now and allowing himself to become even more vulnerable, Jeff pleaded, "Hannah—all my fantasies are about blow jobs. I jerk off in the shower thinking about you doing it to me in college. Part of the reason I fell in love with you was due to our sexual compatibility. I've already compromised quite a bit when it comes to frequency. Trust me, I have other wild fantasies too, but this one is steady and essential. Can't you try overcoming whatever is a turnoff? I just can't imagine life without this. I can't imagine life without you either," he ended glumly.

Technical Instructions

Hannah and Jeff were hoping for a ray of light to shine on their dark mood. I reassured them we would take it step-by-step.

First, Hannah didn't want Jeff to come in her mouth and feared he wouldn't be able to stop himself. Early in a relationship, both parties might not have enough experience to stop before climaxing. Maybe back then, she didn't know what his penis felt like just before he came, and maybe sexual relations were so intensely erotic to him that, being less experienced, he couldn't warn her. Things could be different after several years.

Jeff also needed to tell Hannah if ejaculating in her mouth was an important aspect of the experience he wanted, or whether that simply topped it off.

"I don't think that even ever happened," he said defensively, "but if it did, then either I didn't know she would hate it or I couldn't help myself, like you said. But I know I can stop now. I'd mostly like it if she were just relaxed and natural about blow jobs. I would like to come in her mouth, but when I'm that excited it probably doesn't matter that much."

For the time being he was willing to accept a less than complete fantasy for more oral time.

"And I probably know what his penis feels like just before he comes: really hard and tense. His breathing nearly stops right before orgasm too," Hannah conceded.

Clearly they knew each other better now than in their early time together. Sexual experience can make things easier, but often lovers have written off certain sex acts because of earlier assumptions. One man I know never gave his wife oral sex because when he did, she made horrible faces. Only after talking about it and having her explain that her face grimaced uncontrollably when she was near orgasm did he attempt it again. She had to assure him that he had been so good at it that she nearly came on the spot.

"Okay, but what about the smell and the taste? Even if he doesn't come, I hate the taste of the early drops of semen too."

Jeff could take a shower before sex. And he might try using baby powder around his scrotum. Areas where skin rubs on skin develop stronger odor, like underarms. Anecdotally, I've heard women say they like the scent of baby powder more than that of aftershave.

Hannah said, "Yes, absolutely, I'd want him to take a shower before any oral sex. I just didn't want to tell him and hurt his feelings."

The Taste of Love

As for improving the taste of giving oral pleasure to a man, a woman has a number of options. Here are "Seven Ways to Sweeten a Blow Job":

1. Use lots of saliva to dilute the taste.

2. Stroke him with your hands to further dissipate any leaking semen.

3. Try a commercial product carried in adult specialty stores to add flavor and make it easier for you to maintain a lot of saliva. There are many such products, and one that seems a favorite tastes like Doublemint gum.

4. Hold an Altoid or other strong breath mint in your mouth to salivate more and so that the smell overpowers your own nose. Some men can feel some of the menthol, which they enjoy.

5. Rinse first with mouthwash: we can smell our own mouth bacteria after a bit of time as it mixes on the skin.

6. Drink wine before, during, and after.

7. Request that he refrain from eating strong-smelling foods like asparagus or onions for a couple days beforehand.

Hannah agreed to try these things. She then pointed out that it takes so long to give a blow job that her TMJ gives her jaw pain. The next step, then, was to ask Jeff whether he liked oral sex as part of foreplay or whether he usually wanted Hannah to do it until he's ready to come.

"Both! If she just did it briefly, but a whole lot more often—I'd feel great about that. Every once in a while I'd like her to give me a full blow job, maybe when she's on her period and doesn't want sex but I do."

As we've seen, women, on average, need at least twenty minutes of direct clitoral stimulation to have an orgasm, every time. Some men might also need that much time to orgasm from fellatio. That's quite a bit of oral work. It might be that Hannah was used to him as an even more youthful lover who came easily with such little effort on her part that, later, twenty minutes seemed like a long time. Women can learn to use their hands to provide most of the pressure and stimulation, and their mouth more as an accompaniment near the tip. And women with TMJ might choose days to offer a blow job when their TMJ is at a minimum. Remember, your hands can help stop the man's penis from getting so deep in your mouth as to cause gagging.

Hannah admitted she might be lazy in expecting Jeff to be the giver, and not her. She agreed that she could use her hands, but "that feels like cheating."

With growing hope, Jeff intervened. "Any combination you want to try, I'm up for, Hannah. I wouldn't think you were short-changing me."

Hannah had one final objection: "What about stray hairs? It just ruins it for me when one of his hairs gets in my mouth."

That was certainly going to happen from time to time. Jeff could run his fingers through his pubic hair and tug slightly—called a "French comb"—when he gets out of the shower, in addition to vigorous towel drying that would help get rid of any loose hairs before the action starts.

Slowly, Hannah was able to reintegrate oral sex into her repertoire, giving her a way to please Jeff even when she wasn't particularly in the mood for mutual pleasure, and she eventually came to derive personal pleasure from watching him get turned on.

Let's Make a Deal—or Not

Don't let your negotiating over sex acts break down to horse trading, as in, "I'll do this, if you do that." Trades and scorekeeping reduce the feeling that someone is giving to us because they want to. We want someone to give us a gift because they love us, because they believe it will delight us. Sexually, we want someone to touch us in special ways because they love the way our body responds. We can delight in our lover's response even if we are not personally turned on by doing the specific act.

Remember when you were eleven years old and someone explained French kissing and you thought, "Ew, gross! I'm never going to want someone to stick their tongue in my mouth!"? For some women, the idea of fellatio gets stuck in their minds, recreating the same responses they had when they were prepubescent.

But we can grow to accept—even if not fully enjoy—oral sex in much the same way we eventually develop a taste for avocado or sushi or beer. At first the textures and tastes are too strong and unfamiliar, but over time and with repeated exposure, we become more adventurous.

With regard to oral sex, a step-by-step breakdown of the resistant feelings, countered with tangible solutions, sometimes allows a person to embrace the act and enjoy it. Usually every complaint can be mitigated by some small change or adjustment in the oral sex routine.

Many women talk about feelings of insecurity in their performance: are they doing it right? After another client of mine viewed an instructional film on giving oral sex, she reported, "Everything I saw was something that I had already tried, and that was reassuring. The primary difference between me and the woman on-screen was enthusiasm." A man can reassure a woman by talking or by being noticeably louder when she hits the mark. Jeff thought that suggestion was needless and ridiculous: "Oral sex is sublime, period. Everything about it feels good." But he was willing to try it.

'Tis Good to Receive Too

Women can have negative feelings about receiving oral sex. Renée, a finance manager in a local scientific research firm, could reach orgasm only through cunnilingus. Her husband would gladly perform oral sex each and every time, yet she wouldn't let him. She admitted she liked orgasms, but they were "so much trouble" that she could live without them.

"Why can't Andrew be satisfied with intercourse and let it go?" she asked in an early session with me. She'd sought me out for her low libido, and yet . . .

In fact, she went on, she didn't want sex much at all, though she was willing to do it. I told her that having orgasms would help increase her desire for sex. And then she got to the heart of the problem.

"I can't believe that he would want to do that to me. It's disgusting. He would smear his face in me if I'd let him. I don't understand it, so I can't relax."

So oral sex felt good to her, it brought her to orgasm reliably, and her husband desperately wanted to do it—but she still didn't want him to?

Nodding, she admitted, "I can hear how crazy that sounds when you say it, but yes, that's right."

Why is cunnilingus disgusting? I questioned.

"I think that's fairly obvious," was her simple response, but I asked her to tell me anyway.

She screwed up her face and pulled a shoulder back. "It smells down there. I'm dirty."

Was it her husband, Andrew, who told her that? Did he say it smelled down there?

"God, no!" Renée protested. "He smells my underwear before he throws it in the laundry. But there was a boyfriend before Andrew who wanted me to wash before he'd do it. And I suppose my mother told me I was stinky as a little girl . . . Frankly I think I'm stinky as a big girl."

Ignoring the "stinky" reference for the moment, I homed in on her prior relationship with the boyfriend. Did she let him perform oral sex on her?

"I was really young and less inhibited back in the day. I was also probably drunk when he did it."

It seemed that Renée liked oral sex when she didn't think too much about it. Did she have a higher libido back then too?

"Yeah, I did," she answered with some reservation, seeming to fear the changes that lay ahead.

It can feel like an arduous task to work through anxious feelings that have settled into concrete over time. While we may not like circumstances as they are, changing can be a fearsome challenge. In a more uninhibited state, Renée could enjoy oral sex. And having regular orgasms made for stronger libido.

A few sessions later, Renée was ready to act and asked for my exercises that might change her feelings of disgust. Women's most common anxieties around receiving oral sex focus, as they do with giving fellatio, on cleanliness, smell, and taste. Sometimes women also report that their partner's technique could be better or is too rough.

You Smell Great

A woman's vaginal secretions are clean. If you shower daily, then your genitals do not harbor harmful bacteria. Vulvar odor ranges from mild to strong depending on where you are in your menstrual cycle. Rinsing your labia with water is quite enough to wash off the day's secretions. Sweat glands in the vulva cause more pungent odor than the actual vaginal secretions of a healthy woman. Use soap on your pubic hair and anus to clean away any sweat and bacteria.

I asked Renée to try a test. She was to sniff her underwear every time she urinated in order to notice how her smell changed throughout the month. Sometimes there was a scent like Bradford pear blossoms (seriously), and at other times the odor was a rich and earthy musk. I asked Renée to tell me if she ever thought the smells were unpleasant when she tried this. I have never had a woman come back and say that she smells bad, fishy, or stinky once she has actually tried the experiment. Renée was no exception.

By and large, men do not smell as keenly as women do, plus when they're aroused, their sense of smell is dulled. And while it's difficult for some women to understand, many men love the way a woman's vulva smells and feel very turned on by it. It's not merely that they enjoy giving pleasure, but they feel cheated when a woman denies them access to her genitals.

Renée shared that she didn't like her husband kissing her after he gave her cunnilingus because she found her own taste unnerving. Very brave women can be challenged to actually taste their own secretions. The taste of a woman is often so light that it can be barely perceptible. But a woman smells herself mixed with a man's mouth bacteria and thinks that defines her taste. Asked what his wife tasted like, Renée's husband answered, "Nothing."

"I think the whole issue of fear of our own odor might have to come down to trusting that our life mate is not lying to us," says Susan K. Perry, author of *Loving in Flow* in a personal communiqué with this author. "When a man says he likes it, even if we don't get how that can be, let him have what he likes. It's easy enough to lie back and be generous. Forget the old boyfriends. Some are so fastidious as to be strangers to passion. Phooey on them. Don't let their uptightness ruin the present relationship."

She Knows What She Likes

Receiving oral sex can be uncomfortable if the technique a man uses is clumsy and he becomes defensive when told. Renée's husband would vigorously suck her clitoris when she approached an orgasm. She told Andrew that it hurt but he dismissed her comments, saying she was too sensitive and adding that he could tell she enjoyed it. In a joint session with him present, we were able to help him understand that when her climax was imminent, any continued stimulation would push her over the cliff to an orgasm, but that she was the expert on what felt good. Women reading this might think Andrew boorish, but male anatomy doesn't respond if it doesn't feel good. And hardly any skill is necessary to make his penis feel wonderful. It's impossible for a man to know the best touch for a woman on any given day because a woman's genitals change during the month because of hormonal influences, feelings of energy, clothes she's worn, and the amount of breeze in the air. With specific, direct, intimate feedback, a man can always become more expert and increase his wife's desire for oral sex.

A man isn't a failure even if nineteen of the twenty techniques he knows don't work on a particular night. It means nothing at all about him. "Success" in this intimate realm is mostly beyond reason, beyond practice, and beyond proficiency. It's her body. She knows what feels good and should be encouraged to speak up.

Help Yourself

1. What acts of love has your partner asked for that have made you feel anxious?

2. How frequently do you or your partner prefer to have oral sex?

3. Are there feelings or thoughts that get in the way of your offering oral sex or any other sexual act more often?

4. What have you tried, what are you willing to try, and what are you not willing to try, to please your mate sexually?

5. Speak to each other about oral technique. Name several specific things you like and don't like, perhaps listing techniques and giving them personal number ratings to clarify preferences.

· **CHAPTER FIVE** ·

The Chore Wars

Few things complicate a relationship more than when a couple becomes a family. Children—and for some the conceiving thereof—add entirely new dimensions to a couple's dynamic. Along with the wonder and beauty of becoming a parent, for some the added role complicates the existing marital bond and often the marital bed.

Bree, forty-one, decided late in life to have children. She'd gone through several sexual-intimacy-impairing cycles of infertility treatments over many long years. Having your basal temperature determine when to have sex is not at all like being aware of desire. Infertility treatments can reduce sex to a contrived act devoid of romance and excitement. It can strain relationships over who's to "blame" for the infertility, increased medical appointments and expenses, the disappointing wait for pregnancy, super-hormones, and grief over miscarriages. Baby-hopeful couples might not have sex when they're in the mood if it compromises his sperm count and then again be forced through the motions another night without the spark of desire. Unfortunately, these couples often lose their sexual excitement and spontaneity to the medical mechanism designed to help them get pregnant.

Bree certainly felt like it was all worth it. But now that she had her two very-much-longed-for twin boys, feeding, bathing, diapering, doctoring, and tending them took everything she had. Like many mothers, she couldn't find a way to put an end to her day. She was beginning to measure her success in this new role by how picked up the house was and how often the boys wore collared shirts. And with a dash of perfectionism, her unrealistic expectations had piled sky-high. Exhaustion extinguished the fantasy of growing closer with her husband through their joy as parents.

Originally, Bree's idea had been to stay home with her preschoolers and run her own business on the side. She wished someone had warned her how often kids would be tugging at her for drinks and snacks, because things had not gone according to plan. And she felt constantly guilt-ridden: when working, she wasn't available to the children, and when attending to their needs, she missed deadlines right and left.

Bree's marriage had been crammed somewhere between, or behind, these two other pressing priorities. Sex, by now, had slid far off the plate. When she came to see me, she said, "It's laughable to even imagine that I was once hot to trot. Whatever spontaneity wasn't killed by sperm counts and sex-according-to-my-ovulation sonograms, the babies sapped during their first years. There is no such thing as personal space for me either. By ten o'clock,

I've been tugged at so much I think I'll scream if anyone else touches me." When the kids were finally in bed, sleep was her only priority.

Her husband was unhappy over their lack of sex. Bree expected him to accept the same bargain she accepted: a few disappointments for the incredible gift of children. She described how nothing could ever match the way she felt about them, and added, "Maybe it's wrong—and I do love my husband—but I feel this ferocious, primal love about the kids. They are little for only a heartbeat! And any adult has got to understand that." Her voice breaking, she concluded, "I don't know how to solve this. Money is tight, and I'm so busy I could cry. You asked what I want. I want sex to stay on the back burner for a few more years."

To Do: Have Sex

Sex, as happens in many new families, was now relegated to the to-do list. For Bree, what was once the refreshing pleasure of love-making now seemed another chore. She was tired. She was giving huge amounts of physical nurturing to her family. After an exhausting day of meeting the needs of small children, mothers often complain of being "touched out." Her husband's requests for sex seemed insensitive to her drained feelings of physicality. To get excited about sex, she was going to need structured pockets of time all to herself to recoup her personal space—time she just didn't feel she had.

Bree's maternal nature led her to single-mindedly focus on the children to the exclusion of her husband. For some women, integrating the mother part of herself with the sexual part of herself is challenging. She or her husband could mentally split in two the good mother from the bad sexual object. Chaste, pure, virtuous, and unsullied by selfish desires, the "madonna" cannot experience selfish, sexual fantasies. Often the sexual part, the "whore," is relegated to the carefree, irresponsible days when, with a bad, selfish, lusty, sexual appetite, she was not ready or capable of being a mother. Known as the "whore-madonna" split, this is another reason we later get uncomfortable telling our children about the facts of life; in our culture, virtuous mothers aren't supposed to know anything about sex. Integrating these two parts requires recognition of the problem and a conscious decision to nourish the sexual woman with time and priority.

As it turns out, Bree's instincts were actually leading her astray. By neglecting her husband, she was jeopardizing the stability of her family. I'm not suggesting that sex be used as a tool to "keep a man," because obligatory sex absolutely shreds marital harmony. She needed sex, for relief and play too. And today, with divorce rampant and a child's welfare optimally served in a two-parent household, focusing on the marital relationship by prioritizing time together and intimacy is essential for both partners, and therefore for the children. The boughs of the family tree hold the nest. But no matter how well feathered it is, if the boughs break, the nest will fall.

Healthy intimacy between Mom and Dad is an important gift to give your children. Your model teaches them how to give and take in a loving relationship, providing an imprint for their future intimacy. Distracted, "get-it-over-with" sex is no mother's wish for her daughter's prospective sex life. And because a child particularly identifies with the same-sex parent, low libido may become a female legacy if a daughter senses that Mom doesn't enjoy being the object of Dad's desire.

Even with her best intentions, Bree couldn't remain ever giving to her children without any "me" time. And her business was still developing and demanding.

Here are some suggestions I share with clients like Bree for keeping the fire burning while raising kids:

- Prioritize adequate sleep and exercise for Mom to increase her well-being and productivity.

- Consider a gym membership that offers child care.

- Establish a "quittin' time" after the kids are in bed: no more chores or work.

- Set prekindergartners' bedtime between 7:30 and 8 P.M. Master the bedtime ritual with firmness and repetition. School-age children should be given "room time"—meaning family time is over and they have to be in their bedroom—beginning early enough for Mom and Dad to have some quality time together.

- Set aside four hours of alone time for Mom on the weekend—no kids, no errands.

- Plan a date night that remains unbroken unless the children have fevers.

- Network with other mothers for playgroups, babysitters, community resources.

- Glean a list of good babysitters from known sources in the neighborhood and houses of worship.

- Become comfortable enough with a babysitter or nanny—or extended family member—that you can take a few parents-only weekends away.

- Decide, with your partner, how to fairly divide household chores. If you are a stay-at-home mom, remember that child care is a full-time job; household management is another and should be divided fairly.

- If you are a stay-at-home mom with small children, agree that from the time your partner walks through the door until the children's bedtime, it's "all hands on deck."

- Hire out as much work as your budget and your own schedule allow, including housework, lawn service, bill paying, grocery shopping, and errand running. Hire a college student or housekeeper to do the laundry and start dinner three nights a week.

- Arrange once-a-week lunch dates or before-work coffees with your spouse as a second touch point in the week.

- Take baths together once a week after the kids are in bed. No iPhones, no TVs, no iPads, just relax and talk. Sex optional.

- Get the gift of touch that doesn't have to be reciprocated. Suggest having one evening devoted to getting a massage with no expectations of giving anything back.

- Take the money and time you've been spending (or would have spent) on therapy and continue the investment for child care and a hotel room even once a month.

Bree took my advice and found herself much happier. "No, the laundry didn't run off with the dishes," she said, laughing. "But my children and my husband are more cheerful. And I suppose I might be more productive during the day knowing that an end is in sight. I take almost every night off after the kids are in bed. And I've hired a nanny for every afternoon and my productivity went up immediately, so I can now afford her. You were right, Laurie, I can't be in two places at once. I've stopped preparing and started living."

Sex, for Bree, was no longer a fretful transition between chores and sleep. Now she had the time she needed to connect with her husband so she could feel more sexual. She concluded realistically that her business wouldn't be able to grow as fast as she'd originally hoped until she made enough to hire a manager. In fairness, because her husband's profession was currently more time-inflexible, he agreed to use his vacation time to give her some time to solidify her business. Bree also segmented her home-work hours from her home-family hours. During the evenings, she focused on being really present with them in one short daily play-time and for the bedtime ritual. As she put it, "I'm choosing sanity." And her marriage.

Choosing Martyrdom Is Not the Answer

"All too often, when a man does housework it's a favor," writes Patricia Love, expert on marriage and sexuality and author of *How to Improve Your Marriage Without Talking about It*. "When a woman does housework it's forgotten."

But for Audrey, there were no favors. During her engagement, she came to me already struggling with asserting herself in the relationship. Living with her fiancé, Daniel, she had noticed that he liked to read the paper in the evening while she cooked dinner and cleaned up. She had drawn up a list of what needed to be done around their condo on the weekends; he had dragged his feet about joining in. Lacking much initiative socially, Daniel let her make any social plans, happy to be surrounded by her friends. After their first child was born, she came back to therapy. Things between them were worse.

Both worked full-time but Daniel let her pick up the baby at child care, feed him, bathe him, put him to bed, and do it all over again in the morning. "I get off work earlier, so it does make sense," she justified to me.

She did the grocery shopping and cooking. She also cleaned and decorated their new home. Each took their own car in for repairs, and a gardener did the mowing. But Audrey kept the calendar of all appointments, ranging from her son's well-baby checkups to her husband's dentist appointments. During the holidays, she did all the cooking, all the buying, and all the wrapping. Bill paying and checkbook balancing belonged on Audrey's turf. The weekends also continued to be hers to plan except for the Sunday sports bonanzas. Daniel needed a day of recuperation in order to face the week, she explained on his behalf. So she kept their son busy while he relaxed. Did she have Saturdays to relax and do her own thing? No, that was their family day.

I could guess why she came back to see me. Her sexual desire was nonexistent and her husband found that intolerable. Audrey repressed her resentment. She had no idea that her libido was locked inside the tower of a chore prison. She thought she just came to see me about low sex drive.

More than any other single issue, I see young women's desire drown in the swamp of resentment over an unequal division of household labor and child care. Audrey's situation wasn't an exaggeration, and some women tolerate even more. This is a battle that has to be fought and has to be won in order for the sexy mama to reemerge. According to Gina Ogden, feminist guru and author of *The Return of Desire,* a lot of women don't need more foreplay, they just need "fair play" in sharing life's load. Then desire returns.

I asked Audrey what she had done about evening out the workload. "Whenever I get fed up enough to speak out, he claims that he works more hours and that's true. But as a physician's assistant, I make about fifty percent more money in my forty-hour week than he does even with overtime. I don't rub that in because I don't want him to feel bad or like I'm keeping score."

Losing my therapeutic neutrality, I burst out, "Keeping score? If you kept score you'd explode at this point! And perhaps you need to! Do you ever say, 'THIS ISN'T FAIR!'?"

"I've tried," she replied in a weak voice.

Rather than harnessing her resentment and directly expressing her rage, she had effectively bounced it onto me while she remained pitiable and ineffectual. I was now filled with anger at this ridiculous lack of equality, and somehow she felt better. Unfortunately, this was a familiar strategy for Audrey. All her girlfriends felt the same way about her situation. She'd tell them too about how much more work she did in comparison with her husband, upsetting and agitating them. But she never really fought it out with Daniel. She met her friends' arguments and suggestions with counterarguments. "Yes, but Daniel's sensitive and will think I don't respect him as a man if I bring up the income discrepancy." "Yes, but like he says, the baby really can only be comforted by me." "Yes, but if I ask him to do something, he does it so sloppily, I end up doing it myself anyway." "Yes, but . . ." And so on.

Audrey was emotionally masochistic—she found it strangely rewarding to see herself as a victim of unfair circumstances. Many women would have left Daniel by this point or perhaps not even married him to begin with. Trading her martyrdom for full rights in a relationship was somehow terrifying to her. Here was a woman not limited by economic dependency, religious convictions, or fear of violent retribution by an abuser. Her husband was simply a man who thought it was his due to be taken care of this way. And since she had begun like this, she was afraid that standing up to him would jeopardize the relationship.

To some degree, she was right. It might even take separating to get Daniel's attention. But unconsciously, her lack of desire was saying what she was unwilling to spell out as the issues. In a way, she'd already left him.

I absolutely understood why Audrey didn't want to have sex with Daniel. And maybe he didn't deserve sex—although a sexual exchange based on what we "deserve" is the antithesis of lovemaking. When sex is reduced to quid pro quo, it has lost the very erotic quality that makes it worth doing. If they had come in as a couple, I'd certainly have spent time analyzing Daniel's gross assumptions. Audrey had hoped I might diagnose him as being narcissistic, selfish, or just plain immature, a man with a Peter Pan complex. But a diagnosis that put all the blame on him would mean the situation was hopeless, and I didn't believe it was. There were changes

Audrey could make. Her resentment could be diminished by helping her find a stronger voice.

Don't Be Angry, Be Clear

Another client of mine could never quite understand why she couldn't get her husband to help around the house until she lost her temper. There were two adults in a family. Why should one have to point out laundry that needs doing or mouths that need feeding? But everyone comes with a unique set of assumptions about the structure of a family.

Generations back, it was unthinkable for men to do "domestic labor." Men made all the decisions about money as well. But even today, families with two working parents are often still structured in those traditional ways. Even men and women with feminist sensibilities can fall into roles that might have been defined a certain way in their families of origin but no longer make sense in their modern situation.

It's mysterious why people don't automatically see the needs around them or why they have expectations that are different from each other. But they do, of course. "Men often say they don't see the point of cleaning as much as their wives do," Susan K. Perry, author of *Loving in Flow*, relayed in an email to me: "What looks like an intolerable mess to some individuals may seem casual, relaxed, and homey to others. Such differences may come directly from one's own family of origin, though sometimes two children will turn out the opposite. One may react to a very neat home by copying it in adulthood, while the other rejects it, or is simply oblivious to it while growing up." The same goes for parenting. A woman may feel she needs to imitate her own very traditional and doting mother, while a man may be more passive if his own father was that way.

Caitlin Flanagan, in an essay titled "The Wifely Duty," explained another reason for many women's inability to demand fairness, even though our culture has begun to favor equal partnerships over traditional role-based arrangements. "What we've learned during this thirty-year grand experiment is that men can be cajoled into doing all kinds of household tasks, but they will not do them the way a woman would . . . They will, in other words, do as men have always done: reduce a job to its simplest essentials and utterly ignore the fillips and niceties that women tend to regard as equally essential. And a lot of women feel cheated and angry and even—bless their hearts—surprised about this."[1]

So maybe it's not that he doesn't do things around the house but that he doesn't do them *your way*. In order to sustain a passionate relationship, you need to make your requests crystal clear. From that point, negotiations about who does what have just begun.

Women don't run for election to be the family directress and often don't want the job. But sometimes they have strong opinions about how things should be done. This makes them president by default. Equitable division of labor means moving out of the Oval Office. Women must relinquish control over how often the dog hair gets vacuumed or how organized the linen closet stays. Fathers too have their own ideas about dressing children that may have to be tolerated in a spirit of cooperation. He may do it his way and you need to determine if that can be good enough. What's more important: clothes folded your special way or a relationship that is equitable, respectful, and enjoyable? The goal is to share time and responsibility as a team in ways that maximize each partner's strengths, and free the pair as far as possible for equitable rest, relaxation, and refueling. When a gross discrepancy in responsibility is obvious, it doesn't do you, your relationship, or your sex drive any good to ignore it.

His Mother's Little Prince, but Not Yours

Back to Audrey and Daniel: Daniel's mother had done everything for him. She'd spoiled the baby-king so thoroughly that he didn't know any other way to be. Apparently, in Audrey, he had found someone who would continue catering to him. No matter what she insisted he do, like feed or change the baby, he would leave it for her. And she would do it!

"Well, of course I have to do those things. Our son needs to be fed, and if I don't change his diaper he'll get a rash. I can't let the baby suffer just because Daniel is a jerk." Audrey looked at me as if I were crazy for ever questioning her actions. "Look," she continued, "if I don't do everything, nothing would get done."

I asked her if she wanted to do all the parenting alone forever? The boy would grow too, I reminded her. Someday his father would have to set limits about leaning over the banister or toddling into the street, not to mention dealing with the teenager who might test the limits of alcohol and driving. Even if they divorced, Daniel would have visiting rights and would then be responsible for all the diapers and all the meals.

I suggested she try running some errands outside the house

while leaving the baby in Daniel's care. In fact, my standard suggestion for mothers who are sure their families won't survive a minute without them is to go away for the weekend without any preparation and let their spouses struggle to get meals ready, go shopping with hungry infants, and keep the house in some semblance of order. Absence may not make the heart grow fonder, but it always fosters appreciation.

Still, Audrey had an answer for everything. "If I go away, I will just come back to a bigger mess that will require me to clean up before the next workweek. There won't be any laundry done and the kitchen will be a train wreck. And trust me, if I divorce Daniel, he'll just park at his mother's and let her take care of the baby."

Exercising her autonomy seemed nearly impossible for Audrey. Being needed in an absolute way ensured her place in the world. She depended on her martyrdom, but she couldn't see that. Daniel was dependent, she argued, not her. When I urged her to start confronting him, she balked. She had zero hope that anything would change and she was scared of the huge blowup that would happen if she demanded equality. Instead, she continued to reason with Daniel, explain to him, nag him, and develop lists for him—only to be passively ignored—resulting in a dormant libido.

The Plot Thickens, the Marriage Bond Thins

In the meantime, Daniel started to creep closer and closer to having an affair. He spoke frequently to Audrey about an attractive coworker of his. As a salesman, Daniel took overnight trips, and the next one was in this same woman's territory. Audrey insisted to me that he could not survive without all the things she did for him and would never have the gumption to end the marriage, which she claimed she would do if he cheated. I suspected that these two were playing emotional "chicken."

Audrey was the first to withdraw her demands. The more her husband seemed interested in this other woman, the less interested Audrey became in confronting him about household tasks. Therapy became an urgent place to examine her dependency needs that interfered with her erotic needs. Staying locked in this dynamic enabled her to feel righteous. She was the good mother providing for her child and "husband-son," doing everything for everyone, while she suffered silently.

Rather than demanding sexual satisfaction and fidelity, Audrey now seethed with open resentment. In denial, she began to fantasize out loud that perhaps this other woman was an answer to a prayer—a concubine to satisfy her husband's animalistic needs. I, on the other hand, imagined the affair as a desperate, unconscious attempt on her husband's part to break them out of their "mother-son" pattern. If he cheated, she might get impassioned as the betrayed wife, putting herself in the role of intimate partner. But I knew Audrey's resultant hurt and rage also might forever destroy the possibility of rescuing the relationship.

Audrey had a history that made this scenario even more potentially disastrous. In her early elementary school years, her family's life had been happy. They had regular dinnertimes and there was laughter around the table. Then, when she was in middle school, her father left suddenly, apparently to be with his younger secretary. He had little perspective regarding his own flaws and contributions to the state of the marriage, and he blamed Audrey's mother for not appreciating him and the way he provided for the family. After he began a second family with his new wife, he lost interest in Audrey except when it was convenient to have a free babysitter for her half siblings. Her mother progressively faded into more and more profound depression and was barely able to provide a subsistence living for Audrey and her brother. Often Audrey would come home from school to find the house unlit, no dinner made, and her mother sitting alone in the dark. She had lost both father and mother in the divorce.

Audrey's efforts at homemaking were attempts to give herself and her family the perfect home she had lost. Motherhood was also partly an escape. Days filled with lunch and snack time, playtime, and nap time. We can get lost in the routine of childhood, the days before sexual love complicated our psyche and relationships.

Her father's blame, her mother's withdrawal, and her own loneliness formed a stew that kept her simmering in an unhappy dynamic. To confront Daniel might mean she didn't appreciate his minimal contribution of a warm body in the house. She anxiously avoided reenacting her childhood trauma, especially now that the stakes included her son losing daily contact with his father. Though she was the major breadwinner, she couldn't shake her memories of her mother's impoverished existence. In the meantime, though, another part of her was pushing the relationship toward a crisis by rejecting Daniel in bed.

Freud said we push to relive our childhood traumas because we hope to finally have a different outcome. Audrey's education and career ensured against the financial and economic devastation of her childhood. But having a libido would leave her deeply vulnerable to feelings of abandonment and betrayal. She believed she could protect herself from what happened to her mother only by separating from her eroticism. If you don't want sex, you won't be disappointed when your husband no longer wants you.

The Other Side Speaks

Daniel agreed to come to therapy for a joint session before his next business trip. Expecting someone nonchalant about his marriage, instead I found Daniel interested in Audrey and curious about therapy. Though still struggling against showing her anger, Audrey eventually did work up enough courage to tell him about her childhood losses. Moved by her story and tears, and seeing the potential marital breakup before them, he reluctantly admitted his attraction to his coworker and expressed regret at causing Audrey pain similar to what she'd felt in childhood. Audrey's withdrawal of sex had seemed to coincide with the birth of their son, and Daniel talked about his fear of never being the center of her life again. Feeling pushed out of her and their infant son's intimate twosome and being unable to find a meaningful way to relate to either of them, he had become depressed himself. He fantasized about his coworker to feel more alive again.

Couples tell of sex lives that fall apart because of the birth of their children. Parenthood is full of challenges. But I suspect that, for many, the cracks in their erotic and intimate foundation began much earlier and are then stressed to the breaking point by the arrival of children.

Daniel's own father had left the family when Daniel was four. His mother spoiled him as a way to make up for that absence. A father's role is like a set of arms around the mother-and-child unit that protects them from outside interference and fosters their connection. A good father keeps both mother and child close to his heart, especially during the first two years of parenting, and bides his time for a more central part when he playfully calls the child into a world larger than mother alone and his wife's focus broadens again. Over many sessions, I helped Daniel see how his involvement with his son would mean relief for Audrey and make him important to both her and their son again. I further commended his persistence in trying to regain a good sexual relationship with Audrey. I pointed out that this was one way of reminding her that she was more than just a mother to him.

Like a wounded animal, Audrey lashed out at what she saw as my insensitivity. Was I ignoring her vast bitterness over Daniel's sexual demands in the face of his refusal to share the load? At last, the monster of resentment under their bed came roaring forward with a vengeance.

Finally, Audrey found a way. By yelling at me for my insensitivity, she found a safe substitute. She let out her rage. I acted surprised and contrite at my blunder, which she took as further proof of my taking sides. It infuriated her, finally lancing this boil of toxic marital pus. And because I did not withdraw my concern for her just because she was angry, she grew braver at turning her fury toward Daniel.

When they returned the following week, Audrey recounted how, at home after the last session, a huge blowup had ended in angry sex. Trading her masochism for some momentary sexual sadism, she cursed as she mounted him, bit his lips, and crawled naked onto his face after intercourse to demand oral sex. Daniel was beside himself with pleasure at his wife's first fiery return since their son's birth. His reengagement in the marriage turned the pending business trip to his coworker's territory into a nonissue.

Now able to support what Audrey had begun, I asked Daniel to make a list of the household chores in two columns, each column labeled with one of their names. Refusing my assignment and still wanting to be directed, Daniel suggested that Audrey draw up a list reflecting her ideal division. While his response was far from perfect because it still reflected his lack of ownership in the process, at least it was a beginning toward rebalancing their life. Audrey and I both allowed it.

Resentment is the number one emotional killer of sexual feeling. Certainly many men these days do behave in a spirit of fairness. Men do share domestic labor, some doing more than their share in marriages where sexual problems still exist. But for the others who won't or don't, negotiating a square deal is essential for family harmony—and to wifely sexuality.

Help Yourself

1. List all your household management chores (include making appointments, buying gifts, paying bills, investment decisions, yard maintenance, child care if you both work, etc). Assign a time frame necessary to accomplish the tasks and note who does what. Discuss with your partner a fair arrangement of tasks.

2. Examine your schedule for a block of uninterrupted time (four hours preferably) each week that each of you can use for personal development or rest.

3. Make a weekly date night or morning breakfast for only the two of you. Don't break that date. Ever.

4. Find a second potential intimate time for relaxation and rest that cannot be filled with television, computers, work, or children.

CHAPTER SIX

It's All in Our Heads

While relational equality between a couple promotes an at-mosphere that is conducive to sexual exchange, a wom-an's private thoughts can aid or block libido. When you begin a relationship with someone, your body responds to his touch easily and naturally. Sitting next to your date, you feel your heart speed up. His slight pressure on the small of your back directing you toward your seat sends shivers up your spine. Your hand takes on a life of its own when he first threads his fingers with yours in a dark theater. Which film was it? You can barely remember. His initial kiss got you wet. Desire was so physical, free-flowing, and effortless.

When did it stop being effortless?

Sally, a middle-aged homemaker, knew it was time to have sex with her husband, Michael, to whom she'd been married nineteen years, when she felt a certain zing in her body. But that zing rarely happened anymore.

"When Michael and I were dating," she explained, "it was always time to have sex. I remember being in the mood on every date. My body was on!"

Women married for a few years continue to hope for that remembered magic. They wait for their genitals to tingle.

What we weren't taught to expect, though, is that no woman feels these intense sensations in a long-term relationship at a mere touch, except perhaps once in a blue moon. When we're dating or in a still-new relationship, we engage our minds by constantly thinking of our loved one. We fantasize in the morning about the hot date that very night. We prepare for the big event by shaving our legs and putting on pretty panties. At noon, we might eat less than usual so we fit better into our jeans that night. By afternoon, we imagine salacious innuendos to use at dinner. Having put aside huge amounts of time for romance—six o'clock to whenever— we relax with a glass of Chardonnay and are certain that the night holds love.

We feel desire physically. That's the guaranteed result of ten hours of fantasy.

Fantasy's Active Role

Married women with self-reported normal levels of desire, use their memories, imagination, and fantasy to get themselves in the mood for a physical interlude. Actively thinking about sex and how good it typically feels makes them answer "yes!" when their spouse reaches for them under the covers.

Some women daydream to escape a bit of humdrum and use the pent-up sexual energy to initiate sex later in the evening. During sex, women return to favorite memories: being stroked on the beach by the lake, the first time he gave her cunnilingus, his face in rapture while she stroked him. Secret unshared sexual scenes tease her mind and she uses the oomph of a fantasy to propel her toward responsiveness. Dreaming of having an orgasm, a woman rolls over and wakes her husband. Sexual ecstasy may be the result of a lengthy lovemaking session, or it can be the excited response to a very turned-on partner. But often it is the result of an active sexual imagination. Women with a healthy level of desire have delicious sexual fantasies.

Low-libido women, on the other hand, most often say they never think about sex. And yes, it is normal for women not to think much about sex during the busy day of working, errands, or child care. But if normal doesn't translate to happy, something has to shift. In my practice, I often tease that women spontaneously think about sex as often as men spontaneously think about romance. Unfortunately, in marriages with little or no sex, neither spouse gives enough attention to lovemaking and its accoutrements to change the pattern. But even if men do not need a tender setting in order to feel sexual, they can purposely become romantic. Stocking up on cards, small gifts, candy, and bath oils, and putting a star in his calendar on a random date to bring home a surprise can make a man seem to be spontaneously thoughtful. Similarly, with intention, a woman without spur-of-the-moment thoughts of sex can manage that turn-on click by using fantasy to begin arousing her body.

How to Build a Fantasy

Beatrice, married for fourteen years, had struggled throughout her marriage with low libido. When she arrived at my office, we discussed the possibilities of fantasy, and she asked, "Are you saying, Laurie, that I should just add it to my list? Like, 'number five—fantasize about sex.'" With a grimace, she curtly added, "I don't have time to think about sex."

I suggested gently that since she seemed to have resources of time and money for therapy, perhaps she could set aside some time to think about sex.

"You mean, like homework?" She wondered how she might start fantasizing about sex when nothing sounded less interesting, fun-filled, or exciting to her.

Even if you've never developed the habit of using fantasy in your sex life, it's actually not that hard. Here are some idea sparkers:

- Focus on and "relive" a scene from an erotic dream you've had, a sexy movie you've watched, or a love story you've read.

- Think of a sexual experience you've had, with your husband or a previous lover.

- Dream about your ideal erotic encounter, whether passionate and gentle or rough and dangerous (yes, it's normal to fantasize about this even when in real life a woman is always entitled to say no).

- Put yourself back into a time when you looked forward to making love with your husband.

- Let the rack of women's magazines in the grocery line remind you of all your erogenous zones and remember how it felt to have them caressed.

- As you listen to a romantic song on the radio, put yourself into the lover's role. When Rod Stewart sings "Tonight's the night . . ." see yourself in a sexy negligee reclining on the bed as your lover approaches.

- Picture yourself young, bold, and hot—what would you do with all that power today?

Beatrice insisted it had been so long since she'd looked forward to lovemaking with her husband that she wasn't able to get herself to feel at all interested anymore. I asked her to choose a specific day in her past when she felt sexual, and to tell me exactly what she felt.

"At that time—and mind you, I was very young and receptive—I could hardly wait for him to suggest going back to his apartment. My whole body felt on fire when we started to make out."

Good, I told her. Now build the details. Is it a sunny or rainy day? Where did you go before you went to his apartment? What did you say to each other? What was the sexual innuendo? How did you first touch each other when you got to the apartment?

The same woman who was able to tell me every detail of her children's years-ago birthday parties claimed she'd forgotten the particulars of early love. I pushed a little, reminding her that the beauty of imagination is that historical accuracy isn't required. The initial memory is only the first building block toward a sexy story. So you can make up the details: what you wished you had said, how you wished you had touched each other. Storytelling for adults. Let the tale become more sexually explicit the more you think about it.

"And you want me to do this between soccer practice and making dinner?" Beatrice whined at the end of the session, taking her assignment home without much enthusiasm.

At her next appointment, she gave the report I was expecting: she'd had trouble finding a theme, much like when she'd try to write a paper in college. Beatrice was creative and imaginative, and although she wanted to change, she seemed afraid of it. In previous sessions, she'd openly argued with my suggestions, or, more passively, had forgotten or run out of time to complete assignments. The more time we spent discussing sex, the more her conflicts emerged about claiming desire as her own. Sex had been part of the negotiations of dating, not really an end in itself. She'd been coquettish to attract attention. Now married, she had more attention than she could handle.

As Beatrice explored her resistance to my suggestion, she told me that her guilt overrode her pleasure when she remembered being with other men. And it felt disloyal to her husband to use images of them in her fantasies. As a child, she had been caught masturbating by her older sister, who had tattled to their mother. She remembered the stern lecture from her mother about keeping her hands and heart "clean" following the exposure. Early sensual delight became layered with shame. Lying in bed at all had been considered idleness, and so her mother regimented Beatrice's time and kept her always busy. As a result of her puritanical upbringing, Beatrice struggled to see pleasure as a worthy goal.

The Uses of Erotica

Beatrice found it easier to have her mind stimulated by structured fantasies in erotic stories, romances, or sexy movies. At first she had been afraid that she would stumble across material that would "disgust" her when she looked online for sexy films. Sites for erotica made for women by women, however, offer written summaries of all the material to be viewed.

Recent research by Meredith Chivers, a psychology professor in Ontario, Canada, showed that women's physical arousal was swiftly increased by watching all forms of erotica, even when they subjectively did not notice feeling excited.[1] Basically, visual erotica turns women's bodies on but the plot often leaves her mind uninspired. And some women feel visual erotica might be problematic for their husbands or against their moral frame.

Beatrice decided to give visual images a try. At first, though, she felt conflicted about choosing a sexual tale. When her husband initiated lovemaking, he picked the time and set the pace. Directing her own ideas of a turn-on felt naughty, selfish, and alien. As it turned out, letting her own inner vixen arrange the scene resulted in her getting very wet and excited. The risk she took to direct herself triggered pleasurable taboo feelings similar to her premarital experimentation, and she found her arousal easy.

Bookstore shelves hold quite a selection of erotica and love stories. And without leaving home, you can find sexy books or movies to order online. On the Web, you can choose stories at the right level of eroticism for your own comfort level. Electronic deliveries of books to an e-reader are fast, easy, and private. For instance, the popular *Fifty Shades of Grey* by E. L. James has led to widespread discussion about women's sexual desire and has given many women permission to think and fantasize about sex using written erotica. While some suggest that the book portrays women's secret wishes for kink or dominance and submissive sex games, the appeal of the book is more about a woman being the sole object of desire by a man obsessed with her. The intensity of the sexual connection between the protagonists is what makes the sex scenes hot.

Searches can be customized to balance intensity and comfort. For example, Beatrice wanted her fantasies to remain in line with what she would actually do. Like Karen, whom we met in the introduction, she identified with stories about masterful lovers who seduced virginal women and thus freed their innate eroticism. Nearly every romance novel fit the bill.

Beatrice's marital sexual disappointment, perhaps unfairly, centered on her husband's inability to liberate her from her inhibitions. She thought of the man as the sexual king in the relationship and the woman as his handmaiden until his superior knowledge and expertise made her queen. In her fantasies she wanted to be taken, not necessarily by force, but by someone who would aggressively initiate sex and unchain her latent sexuality.

Many women enjoy imagining sex acts that they would never actually wish to engage in. Perhaps being the center of a ménage à trois with two men giving her their undivided attention. Sex with a handsome, compelling stranger during which she drops her inhibitions completely. Even if they identify themselves as totally heterosexual, some women like being turned on by films of lesbian sex. One of my clients, Chrystal, told me, "I think it's the utter sameness and foreignness of lesbianism simultaneously that I find intriguing—two women both turned on. Their bodies like mine, and so different from a man's." Seeing open female lust in other women gets her in touch with her own sexual self.

Sometimes the further the fantasy is from what's familiar, the more excited the woman becomes as she leaves her mundane day-to-day duties and her own (imperfect) body. She transcends reality into another state of mind. My client Madeleine, a short redhead who considers herself overweight, shared that she was tall, slim, and blond in all her fantasies.

A low-libido woman often feels ashamed about her imaginings, or even ashamed of having thoughts at all during sex. She'd be mortified if her partner knew what she was thinking. Terrified at the idea that somehow her sexual secrets might be exposed, she consequently shuts them down. Perhaps believing that she should climax from purely physical friction, she thinks something is wrong with her, that she is somehow broken, when arousal becomes more difficult and orgasm more elusive. But she's not using all the tools at her disposal.

If we believe that being immersed in the present physical experience is best, then are we cheating our partner when our minds wander? To stop our straying minds, we may try to think of nothing, but then our bodies remain cold. Sex therapist Barry McCarthy writes in *Intimate Desire* that erotic fantasies are most useful at the beginning of an encounter for becoming open and receptive and just prior to orgasm for pushing oneself over the cliff. Used in this way, sexual fantasy serves as a bridge between two people rather than a wall that separates them.

Sensation is often blocked until our psyches engage. Some

women cannot turn on no matter how skillful the caressing unless they see a sexy scenario in their mind's eye. Even a powerful vibrator might not work if your awareness is focused entirely on the laundry. Some women are so anxious to get back to their tasks that foreplay becomes something merely to be endured.

Fortunately, our minds are private. While some couples do include fantasy sharing as part of their lovemaking, for others that would be counterproductive. Sharing certain fantasies may induce jealousy or insecurity if your partner feels threatened by his imagined comparison. The point of fantasizing is to be able to make love with excited participation.

"Not everything needs to be revealed. Everyone should cultivate a secret garden," writes Esther Perel, author of *Mating in Captivity*, making the point that autonomy is as crucial to love relationships as sharing, and perhaps even more essential to desire. And sharing sometimes burdens the originator of the fantasy with having to prove how sexy it is rather than enjoying it for herself.

In order to maintain libidinal fuel for yourself in a long-term relationship, putting forth the effort to remember past pleasures or imagine a new, wild sexcapade can refill the tank. And this thinking can be done consciously, rather than simply hoping that desire will spontaneously flit through your body.

The Erotic Other-Self

Suzie had been referred to me by her sister, a former client. Jeans and a T-shirt du jour were her usual costume. This dark-haired, thirty-eight-year-old, stay-at-home mother had been married to Rob for sixteen years. After a few months of therapy for her low libido, she arrived at a session somewhat anxious because we were going to talk about her fantasies. She had previously mentioned that the central fantasy causing her some distress contained actions that she never saw herself actually performing in bed. She was frustrated by her inability to be turned on without this particular daydream running through her head. With it—during masturbation—she successfully reached orgasm "in under two minutes!"

Why did this fantasy repeat itself over and over in her head? She agreed to explore the story line in therapy. Sometimes analyzing these inner movies can provide rich understanding about our unconscious sexual feelings. While women with high libido might gladly be interviewed and talk freely about their fantasies, women short on desire are often long on inhibition. Their husbands may have already asked the same question several times—"Tell me your fantasies"—in hopes of discovering a treasure trove of touches that would release the inner nymphomaniac. But such wives usually dodge the question. After all, talking about your fantasies and thoughts during sex makes you vulnerable. Revealing our mind is being truly naked.

With a new partner, sex is unscripted. Without a sexual past with this lover, you are able to keep your expectations open to whatever happens in the moment. For this reason, intimacy can feel like a better experience, a spontaneous turn-on. The vulnerability inherent in first-time sex—opening up for a new lover—heightens our arousal. So why, later, do fantasies work so well, when you'd think the goal would be to open yourself only to the moment?

Well, the dilemma, when you're troubled by low libido, is getting to the beginning of the moment. The starting *click* for desire usually doesn't sound until you start the internal movie or sound track. If you feel too guilty to begin the fantasy, you never get to the point of wanting sex.

I wanted to explore why Suzie felt guilty about her fantasy. She took a deep breath and began. "My husband is in my fantasy. But the problem is: I'm not. I have to imagine him with a really sexy, other woman, in order to get turned on. I don't know why I always think about this woman, but it's the only fantasy that reliably gets me to climax.

"She's not someone I actually know, but I fantasize about her so often I feel I do know her like a neighbor or a friend. I've even named her Trenna. Basically, she's a whole lot sexier than I am and has big boobs. And she'll do things I won't. This other woman seems to enjoy the whole experience. I imagine myself watching from a closet or the kitchen pantry. I guess I'm a voyeur."

After listening to a few iterations of Suzie's daydream, I realized that Trenna was a stand-in for the sexual part of herself. She split off her erotic self and projected her onto this imaginary desirous, desiring woman separate from her ordinary self. It wasn't that Suzie had multiple personalities or anything close to it. Trenna was a projection of her inner sexy feelings. Trenna's sexy nature sprang from Suzie's erotic core. She was the programmer and Trenna the computer image doing as instructed.

It had never occurred to Suzie that she was the designer of these erotic encounters. She never initiated sex with her husband, and even if doing so would improve her lovemaking, conveying her fantasies to her husband was so beyond her comfort zone that she just shook her head and looked blank when I asked if she had ever dared.

As we talked further, more details emerged about Suzie's

Trenna fantasy. Trenna's aggressive. She wants to consume her partner. Maybe she's even a little angry. Sometimes she bites his nipples or scratches his back. One time she tore his white button-down shirt off. "She's the type of woman I'd be a little leery of," added Suzie. "The woman at the neighborhood cocktail party who argues about a political candidate loudly or who complains at the association meeting. She'd be someone that you wouldn't want to leave alone with your husband too long either. A real tiger."

Did Suzie consider herself a tiger? "I'm a pussycat, not a tiger," she countered, and I pointed out the slight innuendo in her answer. "A pussy not a tiger . . . I just said that, didn't I? I get fucked but I don't fuck anyone. That is too true. I'm always the one who is screwed in a relationship, but I work very hard at not screwing anyone else. I'm afraid to ask for much. Not at work, not with my teenagers, not in bed."

Reminding Suzie about an earlier lover she'd told me about who hadn't liked cunnilingus, I asked her, "You never said to your lover, 'I don't care if you don't like oral sex, go down and get busy because that's how I come'?"

Laughing, Suzie agreed. "God, no! I could never say that! I couldn't even say something like that to Rob. The crazy thing is that Rob would do anything I'd want him to. He'd die to know I had Trenna inside me. I think he'd come as soon as I tore his shirt off. But I'm just not that forward or demanding. And it's not just sexually. It's just not my nature. I guess I don't think I'd be very likable if I asked for what I wanted. I suppose I've been afraid that if I became a tiger in bed, I wouldn't be very likable—except to Rob, who would love it."

With her walled-off sexuality, Suzie had lost the energy and power to make things in her life go her way. But as so often happens, sex therapy means learning to grow as a whole person. The unexpected thing about changing our sex lives is that we end up changing our lives in many ways. Suzie's "nice-girl" attitudes had flatlined her in the bedroom. Fantasy turned her on when she allowed it, and the analysis of her sexual fantasy gave her new confidence in other realms of her life.

Politically Incorrect Fantasies

Some women may resist using fantasy as a turn-on because of the content of their particular fantasies and the contrast between those fantasies with their actual partner. MaryBeth, for example, sat in my office one day talking about her anxiety about sexual fantasy.

Married for twenty-three years, MaryBeth was middle-aged, slightly plump, and definitely covered up—in more ways than were obvious.

"I can't think sexy thoughts, Laurie," she repeated.

"What do you mean 'can't'?"

"I suppose I believe that what I think about is wrong."

"Morally wrong or just wrong for you?"

"Just wrong for me," she clarified.

"Help me understand: do you mean the specific contents of a daydream or daydreaming itself?"

She sighed, was silent for a while, then spoke softly, with a slight stammer. "Uh, I'm a little embarrassed to talk about these thoughts." I gave her some time to build up her resolve and then at last she opened up.

"I married Craig because he was a decent man whom I could respect. When we met at Berkeley, he was already evolved and tender. Why, then, do I think about this old boyfriend who was nothing like him? Tom was basically rough in bed and an asshole the rest of the time. He'd pull my head back by my hair and French-kiss me and keep me in an almost uncomfortable possessive hold. I'd literally have bruises all over my body from where he'd bitten me. Sometimes he'd tie me up, and he slapped my bottom once or twice. Now, when I let my mind go, I always go back to him and then my mind will even add new scenes to what really happened. Craig would be shocked if he knew I think about Tom. We both knew him in college, and Craig jumped in as soon as Tom dropped me. I'm shocked too that I still think about all this. I never told Craig about the sex with Tom, and he never understood what I saw in Tom anyway.

"I remember being somewhat frightened by Tom because he was so wild. But God! The sex was incredible. His energy! His energy was huge. And if I were to be honest, his penis was huge too. I was a little afraid that he'd ram me to pieces. That element of danger and lack of predictability turned me on. Still turns me on," she finished quietly. "See why I say it's wrong?"

MaryBeth felt that her fantasies about Tom and having dangerous sex with him were a betrayal of her "soft and sensitive" husband. Those were MaryBeth's words to describe him and I asked her to clarify what she meant. Looking chagrined, Mary-Beth explained that Craig's penis was soft now, as was his body. Though she hated that such things mattered to her, she found that her body barely responded to him. He, on the other hand, wasn't turned off by her soft and heavy body. She was ashamed of her double standard.

Tom controlled the sex and dominated her, and that seemed masculine and turned her on. He had a hard body, but, more essentially, a hard and exciting edge to him. Whereas her husband was not only soft in his body but had always been soft in his sexual approach. No exciting hard edges. MaryBeth respected who her husband was as a person, but felt conflicted over what she thought should turn her on and what did turn her on.

"Oh, you hit the nail on the head," she declared. "I am absolutely conflicted. I hate that this turns me on. I don't think men should dominate women, but when I think about it in bed, I get horny. Craig is so patient, so generous in bed; he'd touch me forever, but it just doesn't get me going. I solve my dilemma by not fantasizing so I don't get turned on by things that my husband can't provide. The problem is I'm not turned on at all."

Being dominated to the point of submission, which in turn releases her own true sexuality, is a nearly garden-variety fantasy for women. The idea of being shoved against a wall by a man completely out of his mind in frantic lust for her overrides her inner reserve. Like MaryBeth, women shouldn't be appalled by their own fantasies—no matter how far they are from what they want in reality.

Egalitarians in Bed?

Evolved ideas about gender are one thing—but our bodies haven't necessarily caught up with them. We betray neither our principles nor our partners if our minds choose to get down and dirty to enhance our experience of sexuality. Sometimes, especially with couples who concentrate on technical proficiency, sex gets ground down to a smooth but boring façade over time. Sexual stagnation.

MaryBeth felt conflicted that her fantasy was different from her and Craig's current sexual repertoire. She couldn't imagine her husband bringing the same sexual energy to their lovemaking. With a little reading she might have been relieved to know that her sexual fantasies barely registered on the Richter scale of kinkiness. But women with tiny levels of desire don't often seek out sexual literature like *My Secret Garden*, the first of Nancy Friday's many informed tomes of erotica.

The imagination of a reasonably creative human being can come up with a virtually infinite number of sexual scenarios and ideas. Even if MaryBeth hadn't had a past lover who demonstrated a rougher style, she might have found herself fantasizing about an imaginary lover with similar qualities. What we find erotic is basically outside of our control, not that we have to act on it. We can sometimes increase our erotic feelings about certain acts by exposure, and we can learn to find a variety of activities sexy, but it is much harder to erase excitement over certain scenarios.

Whether it is a specific act or a particular mood that we find most sexually exciting, most inclinations are hardwired into us in early childhood, like the kindergarten exhibitionist fantasy of one of my clients, Cara. As a little girl, Cara masturbated while she imagined her fellow kindergartners parading by her naked body as she lay in a hospital bed. At the time she didn't realize the exciting fantasy was sexual in nature—just naughty because her parents always told her nudity was shameful. Now, as an adult, she had a similar fantasy. She was naked again, but this time it was her coworkers watching her—watching her masturbate or watching her have sex through a one-way mirror.

Many of those early influences come from the family and most are not traumatic; nor do we need to judge them as being dysfunctional. Instead, once we recognize them and accept them, we can act in ways that teach our partner about ourselves. If our partner is turned on by whatever we are thinking, we might suggest acting out an aspect of fantasy. Together spouses decide how much could or should be reality. We can use the ideas to jumpstart arousal into a real encounter with our real partner. Or we can just savor them and enjoy them as ideas that ignite our bodies.

MaryBeth decided to tell her husband about how hard bodies turned her on. Without nearly the amount of defensiveness she had expected, he initiated a daily walk with her and sought a urologist for his erectile dysfunction. Bringing down his weight brought down his cholesterol and improved his erections. He told her he loved her as she was, but also said he'd enjoy the way they fit together if she were thinner. He challenged her to get healthy with him. As Craig's discipline and success over weight loss encouraged her, it also gave her a new level of respect for him. At her last session, she told me they had hired a personal trainer for weight-lifting instruction together.

Flesh and Spirit

Brought up in a small town in North Carolina, Alexis had been part of a rural community that was economically depressed and relationally enmeshed. Tall and impeccably dressed in a navy skirt, this lovely, young African-American woman described her home. Everybody knew everybody. Her father had left her mother when she was four but still lived down the street. Her stepfather had been the town's preacher, and ran a strict and structured household. She was currently a deaconess herself in a small church where parishioners shouted amens and held healing revivals. Spiritual exuberance was juxtaposed with moral tautness.

Alexis told me that although she loved her father, there was little to respect about him. He did whatever he wanted without regard for his wife or children. Her stepfather, though "intense," saved the family from poverty and despair. She held him in high esteem for the way he took on five children and gave them a way of life that turned out five decent adults.

Now married, Alexis was a successful small-business owner. She came to therapy because of her lack of sexual interest in her husband. After several sessions, I understood the centrality of her fight between selfishness and righteousness. That conflict represented the difference between her father and her stepfather, with the well-being of her family held in the balance. Pleasure was always suspect for Alexis, and she reacted strongly when I brought up the subject of using imagination as a bridge into desire.

Alexis sat up on the couch. "I can imagine many things—things that soothe me, things that stimulate me—but ultimately both feel wicked to me. Some things don't lead to a productive life."

For Alexis, fantasizing about sex seemed a step down the path to hell. Such thoughts brought to mind her father, who put his indiscriminate liaisons with other women ahead of his responsibilities.

"I don't want to make decisions based on my flesh; I want to be able to have sex with my husband and live according to principle."

Backing off somewhat, I said, "It seems that maybe I've offered an idea that is really off the mark. Tell me what you mean by decisions based on your flesh."

Alexis explained that, in the extreme, she meant drugs, sex orgies, or instant riches—things that corrupt the soul. She believed that using fantasy was too much like a cheap trick when "I should be involved with this man, in this time, in this place."

I reassured her that I didn't want her to do anything, ever, that felt like a gateway to immorality, but she needed to know that a woman's mind has to be involved in her sexual experience. I asked her if there might be some way she could help me help her use her mind in a way that would seem loving and acceptable and not make her feel like she was compromising her morals.

"I confess I've thought of an earlier lover from back home," Alexis began, getting to the real reason she objected to my suggestion. "I've done it and, you're right, I get hot and bothered. The worst thing is that my mind has a man other than my husband fulfilling me and my body craves a man other than my husband. I pray never to go there again. I'm afraid your idea of fantasy would put me on the path to infidelity and sin."

I wasn't about to ask Alexis about her fantasies of the other man. I believed that we could find a fantasy for her that would cue her sexually and be morally acceptable. But I was afraid to explain myself more as she was already so guarded. Her anxiety over the possibility of thoughts leading to temptation was very real for her. But once she admitted imagination had the power to change one's state of mind, I had an idea.

Prayerful Projection

Fantasizing about sex can induce a more relaxed receptivity when your spouse initiates sex. Many things can change your state of awareness to make you more susceptible to suggestion or new ideas. Hypnotherapists directly try to alter a patient's consciousness to make suggestions for change. Drinking, smoking, and drugs all produce altered states, but so do music, worship, meditation, exercise, and prayer.

Acknowledging Alexis's fear that if she relaxed her vigilance and daydreamed, she might be lulled into sinful thoughts, I suggested she fantasize having a sexual and loving exchange with her husband and responding in an excited way. Would it be possible for her to think only of these things, almost a prayerful projection of what she wanted to experience with him?

Alexis considered this carefully. "We do claim many things for the spiritual realm in my church. I think I could do that and not feel like I'm straying from God's teachings. I believe I must make my marriage better and our sexual life is a big part of that."

The contents of your fantasies can align with your morality, though that's not necessarily automatic. Many women in my southern community—even those without a strong, religious belief system—also express concern about the rightness and wrongness of using their imaginations to spark their desire.

Alexis struggled hard to be an upright woman and wanted to find a way to increase her sexual desire without compromising her morals. Indeed, she took her marital vows seriously. Her husband was to be happy and their marriage was to have all the fullness that she had committed to. But her instructions about how to be a whole sexual creature had been incomplete. She had relied on the mood striking her, and given her busy life, that wasn't likely to happen often. Allowing her imagination a bit more leeway made a real difference to her marriage. Pat Love, noted sex therapist and author of *The Truth About Love,* says that "lovers stay connected through fantasy, anticipation or thinking of ways to please one another. These frequent expressions of caring deepen the connection between the two and eventually become part of the phenomenon we call love."

Help Yourself

1. Describe your favorite memory of a date with your partner. Describe the first time you made love.

2. What would be an ideal date? What are three things your partner can say and do on the date to make you feel amorous?

3. Observe the way your environment prompts you to think about sex. Include songs, articles, movies, conversations, and innuendo during the day that have sexual content.

4. Build a sexual daydream. Use a sexy prompt to start a twenty-minute reverie about the best sex you can imagine. Picture the setting. Create explicit dialogue. See detailed sexual caresses. Feel the crescendo.

CHAPTER SEVEN

Seduce Me Like You Mean It!

*S*he glimpsed his taut abdomen exposed by an unbuttoned white linen shirt, brown curls trailing to below his trim waistband. Turning around, she tingled as he came to stand behind her, the length of his body hard and firm against her back. In the evening's waning light, his strong hands began to caress her shoulders and arms, his musky scent faintly tantalizing as he nuzzled her hair. He whispered his desire for her. While his fingertips began to gently trace the sides of her breasts, he told her how she would quiver with excitement when he finally made love to her . . .

Women fantasize sexually about being seduced. Romantic movies and books devote many scenes and pages to building sexual tension. Men who are dating spend money, time, and energy trying to create an experience that will make women swoon and then fall into bed. It's nearly formulaic, an instinctive part of the hunt. Even women who never read romance novels or watch so-called chick flicks long for and enjoy the game of seduction.

The script goes something like this: He's attracted to her. He tells her repeatedly of his desire for her. His sexual energy is on a short leash. He pays homage with his resources to her romantic needs. He engages all her senses: smell, sight, hearing, touch, taste. For a moment in time he conveys that she alone is the most important thing in his world. He moves slowly with confidence. Or using his male aggressive energy he rips her clothes off. He reads her readiness because he's utterly tuned in to her.

Compare this with what passes for seduction sometime later in the relationship: "Hey, hon, you want some nookie in the shower?"

I'm not saying that women don't also need to play their part in this dance of seduction. Nor that women shouldn't be seducers and initiators in the bedroom. Obviously, if a woman never initiates, she gives up control of having sex when she is most ready for it and remains dependent on chance synchronicity.

But a low-libido woman could really use a guy who's an expert seducer.

Sometimes seduction is missing or halfhearted or inept, in which case, male desire simply won't carry the day. Sometimes a woman meets her husband when he's in late adolescence or before he's fully come into manhood and developed a mature style of sexual approach. Maybe his comments are too coarse or too juvenile and so she turns off. Perhaps he lets her know that he's horny, but does this as an undirected feeling, not a flattering solicitation about how she, in particular, turns him on.

At times, women actually discourage their men from being

romantic by their lack of appreciation of or outright scorn at the man's flawed or feeble attempts. Men often complain that they did all that seductive stuff in the past and it didn't work, so why try now? Sometimes women are turned off by a man's obvious fear of rejection and lack of confidence. And certainly, I've seen the resultant vicious cycle held in place by rejecting women who complain that their man's seductive attempts are never quite right.

Most husbands married to women short on libido have heard every excuse in the book. They feel powerless to ignite her desire. Every man remembers a time he brought flowers or planned an impressive date only to be turned down sexually later. And women often complain that he only treats her in special ways to get sex. That makes her feel manipulated. She may say she wants more romance and seduction, but once he begins to act romantic and sexy, she might keep him at arm's length. She's afraid his gestures aren't genuine, aren't from the heart. He only did it because she asked. Of course, not doing what she has asked also proves his lack of love, so it becomes a lose-lose situation.

Talking about their lack of seductive skills can make men, utterly depressed about their low-sex marriage, feel like they're to blame. But the quality of seduction matters. Men need to step up to the plate and take an appropriate role in assertive seduction. Especially during the low-energy years of raising children, male seduction is the way the couple can share testosterone. Unfortunately, as all dynamics in sexual life, it's never quite as straightforward as we might like it to be.

Low-libido spouses who long for more enthusiasm must consider that they might be participating in a vicious cycle that keeps things calm. Perhaps the calmness soothes their anxiety about the post-honeymoon realization that they're different people after all—not the idealized mate they had dreamed of marrying. Or the tranquility of staid, boring sex can result from an inability to withstand conflict. Their apparent serenity hides their feelings of anger and aggression toward their partner because neither is really mature enough to take the heat. Damping down high eroticism and excitement protects each partner from the possible humiliation of being rejected right when they are feeling the most sexually vulnerable.

The woman may unwittingly encourage a flat-footed, nonseductive approach: romantic heroines are not usually dressed in sweats and baggy T-shirts. She too may need to step up her game.

If this cycle of boring or no sex continues for too long, the husband may also shut down.

Excuses, Excuses

Matthew and Jenny were studying in the same masters-in-business-administration program and were planning to form an online company to sell elegant home decor. They'd been living together for three years and had been seeing me for minor difficulties that included sexual problems. They were going to marry as soon as they were financially stable enough to afford a wedding.

Dressed in holey jeans and artfully mismatched layers, Jenny sat beside Matthew, who was similarly attired. With straight brown hair that hung down into his eyes, Matthew radiated a gentle spirit that complemented Jenny's fiery intensity. They had fallen in love during undergraduate art school, and thought of each other as soul mates. She loved his flexibility and he loved her exciting energy.

The main problem that had brought them to my office was that Jenny avoided sex. She used one justification after another, but ultimately felt that her innate passion did not extend to the erotic. At this point, they were having sex once a month, and their negotiations over when and how often spoiled even those few interludes.

Jenny produced an actual list of times sex was absolutely off-limits for her:

When she was on her period
At her parents' house
When any of their parents were visiting
Too late at night
In the morning
During exams
After a big meal
Anytime she felt fat
When either was sick or contagious
During a herpes outbreak (they both had it)
During her favorite TV show
When company was expected soon
If she'd had too much to drink
When their bedroom was dirty
When the dishes were undone
If she hadn't showered
If he hadn't showered

In fact, it's not all that unusual for such libido-killing lists, though rarely written down, to hover in the back of some women's minds. I asked Matthew how he felt about Jenny's list.

"Jenny's a control freak," he said with a sigh. "Really, the list is much more extensive and it includes how I initiate too. She wrote that out one day when I complained that her rejections were completely random and she argued they were patently obvious. Basically, I've stopped approaching her. I love her and I guess I still want to marry her. I'm trying to deal with the fact that sex is going to be entirely on her terms and not very frequent."

Asked when they actually found a "right" time to have sex, Jenny explained that they had it when she felt guilty enough, and that usually took about a month after the previous time.

Matthew shrugged without anger. "It wouldn't do me any good to get all worked up about it. So I wait for when she gets around to it. She says it's a month between, but sometimes it's six weeks or as long as two months."

What If He Gives Up?

Withdrawing sexually can seem like the perfect solution to a man who is repeatedly rejected. And initially the low-libido woman may experience relief. He may choose to masturbate in private. Perverse marital dynamics emerge if she insists he match her lack of desire and resist any form of sexual release. If indeed he acquiesces and kills his desire either as an attempt to prove his twinship or out of his own despair, the odds of getting marital intimacy back on track are poor.

Shutting down is a temporary and treacherous solution. Eventually his desire will resurge with a backlog of resentment that could damage the relationship further. He may find this earlier tacit "partnership-without-sex" agreement too empty for the rest of his future. If that moment coincides with an interested other party, it doesn't take too many sparks to light a fire. Even if he resists an affair, his being wanted often breaks the dam of emotional pain and washes out the remnants of a marriage or relationship.

Jenny further explained the problem from her perspective: "Matthew has bad timing. He never seems to initiate at times that make sense. I give him a look like, 'Seriously? You think it would be great to have sex now while we're rushing to get out the door to go to work?' Or he gets this little-boy smile. I cringe when I see it because I know he wants sex, but it makes him seem like he's fourteen years old! And these days, he doesn't put any creativity into seducing me. I figure, if he doesn't want it enough to do anything about it, I'm not going to feel too bad denying him."

After spending more time with this couple, I wasn't sure whether Jenny genuinely lacked desire, or if she was just very sensitive about the timing of sex. She was certainly resistant. I could see that the initiation phase of their lovemaking was way off. Matthew was too tentative. His defeated attitude kept him from providing energy that she needed. But in his eyes she had contributed to the mystery of their sexless relationship by underscoring what didn't work rather than what did work.

I asked her to describe three ideal times to make love. Surprisingly, she was able to rattle them off.

"Friday night after a glass of wine and before dinner, Saturday afternoon when we've finished running around and have actually spent some time together, and Sunday after breakfast."

Incredulous, Matthew jerked his head up as he turned to look at her. Before I let him protest, I wanted to press my advantage and asked to hear her favorite fantasies of seduction.

"Matthew used to be sexier. When we started dating, he'd do things like caress me in the car on the way home from dinner. He'd make me take off my underwear in the car. Then we'd get home to my apartment and he wouldn't let me turn on the lights but would undress me right in the living room. He'd turn on music and we'd dance naked in the dark just holding each other close. Once he turned on hard-rock music and threw me on the couch and went for it. He can do it; he just doesn't anymore."

Not to be held back any longer, Matthew nearly shouted. "That is so unfair! Do you realize how many of your rules those scenarios would break now? All of them took place way too late at night! After you'd been drinking. And after a big dinner! You were never tired back then. And you say the weekend is a good time? I've tried some of those times and you never want to have sex. And how do I undress you in the dark when none of the times you describe are at night?"

Matthew's anger was much more apt to change things between them than his passive hopelessness. Much of what he said was undoubtedly true. She needed to examine the contradiction between what she currently demanded and what turned her on in the past. Sexual resistance couched as "never being the right time" can be difficult to break through. He did need to push Jenny about her rigidity. Her need to control had pushed sex into a corner. Yet Jenny too did not really want things to go on as they had. She had focused so much on "just the right time" that she really was completely out of touch with any natural feelings of desire. Her rebuffs had stuffed down the very aspects of his aggression that she liked. They were ending up having sex when neither was very enthusiastic.

Whether it was a messy kitchen or bedroom, or whether sex hadn't been tightly choreographed into the routine, her anxiety about minor changes to the schedule and her need for order were greater than average. Maybe even obsessive. I imagined that sexual arousal and exchange felt chaotic to Jenny. She was defending something internally, not just Matthew's advances. Jenny had to work to see that making order her highest value was not actually bringing her happiness. Hot sex demands chaos, lack of control, and surrender. Eventually she came to realize that she would not have a secure relationship—and later a marriage—unless there was good sex. I believed her willingness to change was weakly peeking through in her suggestions for times that sex would be good for her.

Once Matthew had a chance to express his anger and hurt, he needed to examine the ways it had been easier for him to become passive than to fight for intimacy. Matthew had allowed himself to be designated as the sole problem. He avoided conflict because he was afraid that if he pushed her, he'd lose her. Seducing well, though, meant that he had to be his own person rather than simply trying to fit into Jenny's perfect mold. He had been rejected, yes, but his dependency on the relationship was keeping him from expressing his true needs. It was a vicious cycle: the more he accepted uptight Jenny's strict requirements about when to have sex, the less she respected him, the more depressed he became, and the less energy he put into sex and seduction.

Jenny wasn't crazy about what I was suggesting. While she didn't like that Matthew seemed afraid of her, she also didn't like the idea of him becoming more confronting. It was scary to her to see her power slip out of reach. But the reality is, if we can completely control sex, we won't want it. We might as well masturbate because that's what we've reduced it to. (Not that I'm against masturbation—just making a point.)

Seduction Tips

To get him back on the road again, I helped Matthew with advice about seduction. Jenny's memories indicated that she was more responsive to using touch for initiation, while in frustration Matthew had started to clear the way with verbal requests. I offered the following suggestions for turn-ons:

- Tell her how desirable she is—often.

- Remark on the variety of ways she's attractive—sexually, emotionally, intellectually.

- Make sure she knows *she* is the object of your desire—not simply that you're horny.

- Vary your pacing during initiation—whispering, teasing, urgently, slowly.

- Be direct—use a serious, strong voice when you tell her you want her.

- Tease her with your touches; make her wait for explicit touching.

- Use whatever resources you have to make the setting suit her preferences.

- Be romantic: send cards, call during the day, plan dates, bring flowers every so often (make a plan once a year and put it in your BlackBerry or calendar and you're done!).

- Engage her senses: I can't overemphasize how most women like clean smells and fresh breath. Take baths together! Shave. Light candles. Simplify the bedroom to be more like a hotel room than an office or laundry room. Touch her throughout the day, not just when you want sex. Feed her strawberries and champagne. Put music in the bedroom.

- Look her in the eyes before you kiss her.

- Know that desire often kicks in *after* arousal for many married women—she may only really *want* to do it halfway into the experience.

- Give her your undivided focus once a day beyond the bedroom.

- Take her on getaways.

- Be insistent and resilient.

Sex requires effort and planning. During our dating years, we spend enormous amounts of energy getting ready for erotic encounters. Then, in the more settled years of commitment, we want to believe that desire springs spontaneously in the moment. But the dance of the seducer and the seduced needs skillful attention. If forgotten or buried, this tango is relearnable.

A woman disappointed in her partner's efforts has to change her reaction to change the cycle. She has to tolerate some wavering and some anxiety. Owning her right to desire frees her from the need for perfect ministrations. Appreciating his efforts even if clumsy at first will go a long ways toward strengthening his resolve to be a good seducer. Relinquishing the fantasy that real sex should be seamless and require little instruction allows a woman to move into a more mature sexual relationship where she too is at the helm and can direct the encounters to fit her wishes.

Help Yourself

1. What are your favorite memories of seduction? Or favorite love scenes of erotic tension building?

2. What elements of these memories and fantasies are missing now? How have you changed?

3. Ask trusted friends about their perception of your need for control. How does it keep you safe or keep you dull?

4. Find two new ways to risk being open to seduction.

CHAPTER EIGHT

The Birds and the Bees:
Effects of Childhood Messages

I deally, we emerge from childhood feeling loved and safe enough to love back. The sexual legacy begins while suckling at the nurturing breast in complete dependence and symbiosis with mother. The nursing mother helps the anxious infant become relaxed, no longer hurting from hunger pains. If hunger relief comes regularly, then psychologically the child begins to trust that the world will meet her needs. Physical needs become acceptable and the child is able to wait with a growing confidence while Mommy gets ready to nurse or fixes the bottle.

With tender care and constancy, the child differentiates from her mother and begins to see her as a separate being but continues to feel connected to this other who dependably comforts and meets her needs. Inner needs feel acceptable and reasonable. Appreciating mother's separateness happens after years of feeling attached. While the father's (or partner's) role is first to shelter the mother-child couple, he (or she) too comes to play a significant part in creating safety in attachment to others.

Relational hope is the family's gift. With faith in the world to meet our needs, we believe that people will satisfy our intense longings.[1] We don't have to depend strictly on ourselves. When we're depressed, we react by calling a friend. When we're happy, we think celebrating with loved ones will add even more joy. When we're lonely, we reach out. When we're lustful, we seduce our lover. We look to others to feel fulfilled and happy.

Relational hope is necessary for healthy desire. More than simple mechanical functioning, libido is not simply driven by the body or our hormones. In marriage, we must trust the world of relationships enough to allow ourselves this intimate need. Sexual desire for women continues to contain the deep need for emotional attachment to the beloved, argues sexual researcher Rosemary Basson.[2] Feminist theory has broadened our understanding of the psychological gender differences in growing up. About the intimacy and identity stages of development, Carol Gilligan writes, "Instead of attachment, individual achievement rivets the male imagination . . . women, however, define their identity through relationships of intimacy and care."[3] For girls, our eventual identification with our mothers means we do not have to fully sever our ties in order to mature. In fact, connection remains a key to our psychic health.

As we've discussed, men and women alike fantasize about closeness and merging. Both romanticize that someone, like mother, will meet their needs without being asked. Yet even the best mothers, in reality, were never as consumed by the infant as the infant, in its limited knowledge, believed. She had a spouse, perhaps other children, and many friends who also shared her love. But the infant's survival is so dependent on the mother that this separateness is intolerable information in the beginning. When a family is healthy (not perfect, but has provided good nurturance as well as appropriate limits to the naturally egocentric child), the individual grows up confident and secure, ready for the pleasure of merging with the intimate lover of their choosing.

If, however, our parents do not meet our needs, we pick up in childhood that the world is a random or harsh place and we learn that our needs don't much matter. Without plenty of affection and warmth, we will quiet our inner needs. Worse, we might conclude that our needs are dangerous because they make our caregivers angry. So we shut down; we stop wanting. If our caretakers are cold and rejecting, we grow up to avoid close contact, and in adult romantic relationships, we are predisposed toward the distancer side of the continuum. If our caretakers were intermittently chaotic, and there were early separations or only partially met needs, we grow up anxious and ambivalent about connection, and in adult romantic relationships, we lean toward being a pursuer. Even good childhoods have inevitable lapses that direct us toward one or the other side of the closeness/distance dynamic. The closer to the center we are, the more secure our childhoods were, the more flexible we will be in our adult romantic relationships.

Harville Hendrix explains in *Receiving Love* that our primitive longing to be touched and stroked evokes powerful links to childhood memories and how those desires were handled as children. A difficult or lonely childhood often kills sexual passion in the adult.

Parents do not have to be cruel or purposely withholding to

wound a child. Families may be structurally sound and still not provide enough love for a particular child because of life's circumstances, birth order, or a parent's own inadequacy. Perhaps the mother is sick or depressed during the crucial early years of a child's life. Or the last of six siblings is born to older parents who have exhausted their caring years. Children can suffer benign neglect and be given toys, possessions, and entertainment instead of time and attention. Parents may see their duty to their children defined particularly as instructors and teachers and focus dominantly on good behavior, perhaps to the exclusion of exploring and enjoying the relationship with their child.

To become close to another person sexually and to fall in love necessarily draws from our childhood sense of whether we believe we are lovable. We may be Mother Teresa now, but if our parents once said we were selfish, their opinion remains absolute truth. If our parents were too preoccupied or too selfish themselves to give to us, we believed it was our fault. Allowing someone to love us when we do not feel wholly—if at all—lovable challenges the world as we know it. We would rather hang on to the familiar feeling of being unloved than enter a parallel and true world where we are treasured, cherished, and desired. Being loved throws the world out of whack! "Self-rejection is the most universal and least recognized problem in our lives. It is the source of all our difficulties in giving and receiving love," write Hendrix and Hunt in *Receiving Love.*

Whether we are aware of it, all of us need touch and attention, and children will learn to guard themselves from further disappointment in life by deciding that they can live without it. By the time they are adults, this inner vow against needing others has become so cemented into their character they can't remember the reasons for their formidable defense. Women who grew up this way will often tell me that they are just not affectionate people. She distances herself from her lover in order to keep the world as she knows it on its axis. Sex that comes from this distancing stance can be fearful or aggressive. It can be withheld, fail technically, and ultimately is usually expressed as no sex.[4]

The stronger a family's construction, the more it bears analysis. Functional families invite review in order to have everyone's feelings and opinions understood. Questioning in a healthy family doesn't crumble or destroy it. In other, more fragile family systems, scrutinizing the past can feel worrisome. We can be torn by loyalty. Adults from families that avoid examination often shy away from looking too closely. We can be afraid that our seemingly solid foundation might dissolve into sand. Sometimes it's easier to forget about childhood or gloss over it. You might say, "It was a long time ago—what's the big deal?" Sadly, an unexamined history means repeating the previous generation's problems. Maybe not exactly, but certainly in some way. The power struggle in this generation can distill problems inherited from both families, creating an even more toxic brew.

Sexual desire demands capacity to give ourselves over to the hands and touch of another, expecting to receive pleasure and comfort. It requires us to be aware of our need for physical touch in the first place. In this chapter we will explore the historical reasons for low desire not as an excuse, but as an explanation, for our feelings. Once we have found some roots of the problem, we can take steps to remedy the losses of childhood.

Sleuthing through your family's history can yield important clues about your levels of desire—or utter lack of it. What they actually told you about the birds and the bees is not the most crucial aspect of your sexual foundation. That so-called pivotal sex talk is irrelevant, insists Jack Morin in *The Erotic Mind*. "Children absorb what we truly believe through our unrehearsed comments and behaviors." Far more important, the romantic triumph or tragedy of your parents' own sexual relationship shaped your expectations for your own intimate partnership.

We don't witness our parents' life behind bedroom doors, but we do sense it. If their love is strong, we feel sheltered in the boughs of the sturdy tree holding our nest. When their bodies— and moods—are silent or frustrated, we intuit the precariousness of our fragile branch. Parental love, toward each other as partners and toward us as children, creates our later capacity to give and receive love, both emotionally and sexually.

Overt Family Messages About Healthy Sexuality

In a healthy family, our parents' loving, caretaking touch connects our mind to our body. Slowly, we distinguish the outline of our body as our own. Our mother's loving gaze while feeding and rocking us is like soul sunshine. Her loving eyes convey to us that we are good—giving the earliest and deepest basis of self-esteem.

A child-centered schedule teaches the infant that her needs are reasonable. Rather than forcing a child to cry it out, parents take the baby's distress seriously and address it as immediately as possible. Regular cycles of rest, play, and feeding reduce the infant's anxiety.

Gentle diapering without repulsion allows a child to begin to integrate her genitals as her own and as a source of pleasure, not of shame. Toilet training is relaxed and child-driven as the girl masters control of her evacuation functions. No humiliation is expressed for failures.

Early genital self-stimulating explorations are met with her mother's understanding smile and the girl is directed to have these exquisite sensations in private. In early childhood, self-stimulation feels good and is a natural part of growing up. These early experiences don't signify sexuality as much as pleasure seeking and comfort seeking. If parents handle this well, reassuring the child about her delightful discovery—that her body was meant to feel good—the child starts to own pleasurable bodily feelings as powerfully under her control.

Naming a girl's body parts should include accurate distinction of her genitals: vulva, labia, clitoris, vagina, and anus. Tragically, in my work as a sexual instructor, I've learned that the clitoris— the unique female body structure devoted solely for sexual pleasure—is nearly always unnamed by her mother. Along the way we are told about "bad touches" and taught to say no and tell Mommy if someone should try to touch our private parts, in order to protect us from molestation. Knowing actual terms for her vulva and the structures within (clitoris, urethra, vagina, anus) helps protect a girl with accuracy should she ever have to recount a dreadful violation.

Kisses and hugs are given to us every day. Mommy smiles at Daddy when he reaches out to kiss her. We know something electric happens in Mommy when she's dancing with Daddy. It feels good when Daddy tells us we're the most beautiful girl in the world next to Mommy. We see him wink at Mommy across the room at parties.

Even if Mom is single, her eroticism gives her energy that helps her with all the parenting tasks. We feel her excitement about a future partnership. Questions about sex are given straight answers. And our parents initiate the conversation at appropriate ages if we're too shy to express our curiosity.

Our childhood crushes are never subjects for teasing. Being caught in childhood sex play doesn't result in hysteria but is simply corrected with appropriate boundaries and redirection. Unalarmed, Mom says, "Okay, everyone put your clothes back on; clothes need to stay on. Now, we're going downstairs for a snack."

In a sexually healthy family, Mom teaches us all about our period and the way we'll become a woman. She buys us a stash of woman-things for the day it finally happens. She tells us that our bodies will soon be filled with passionate, exuberant sexual feelings and that sex is one of the most exciting experiences in life. Everyone is excited when we start our period, and we know Daddy knows too because he gives us a big hug.

Mom talks to us about excited feelings that come with being with a partner. She tells us it is natural and a wonderful part of life. Both Mom and Dad say that sex is a gift for people who love and respect each other. We talk about how to know when it's the right time for sex, how to tell if we're ready, what that will feel like. Our parents convey their moral and relational ideas about sexuality and listen to what we think as well. If we feel more drawn to girls than boys, our parents respect and support our choices.

Our parents have some rules about what kind of clothes we can wear out of the house and make sure to meet our dates and have little talks about "safe driving" and "valuable cargo on board" with our date. There are limits that confine and frustrate us somewhat. Our parents want answers to "who, what, when, and where?" before we go out.

Mother may be the role model, but father has a special duty too. He sees the beauty in his developing daughters from the lens of protective love and assures the gawky adolescent of her future attractiveness. Girls who feel valued by their dads for their intellect, character, and various talents, as well as for their beauty, grow up with confidence about their interactions with men.

Mom praises us too, telling us how gorgeous we look in our new dress and smiles warmly when we ask her how we look before we go out. Her pride in our attractiveness is not diminished by angst over her own changing beauty.

She reminds us that we must be the one to decide when we are ready to have our first amazing sexual relationship. Birth control is openly discussed.

It's Dangerous out There, Isn't it?

Unfortunately, our society has angst about a girl's development that doesn't pertain to boys per se. Parents fear a daughter's sexual awakening. They worry about pregnancy. And now the media makes every disaster, kidnapping, and tragedy seem like it's happened next door. Rightfully, parents worry about sexual violation. And it becomes easy for parents to focus more on protecting their girl from others than on preserving her sexual core. Even a little girl rubbing herself against the couch can stir up more anxiety in parents than her toddler brother reaching down his pants. There is simply a cultural belief that girls do not and should not own desire.[5] Daniel Steinberg, editor of a collection of writings called The Erotic Impulse, notes that "Girls are taught that sex is their enemy. Sex is a beast, a male beast and it is the female task to tame this beast. Sex contains . . . the danger of destroying one's status among the society of good girls. Sex as pleasure is permitted if it's essentially an expression of love for a partner, but sex for its own sake—lust, desire—is unfeminine." While we may need relational connection to sustain sexual feelings, we are taught that the feelings themselves are dangerous.

First Partner

Transitioning to partner sexuality is a process. Teens frequently use masturbation to make up for the losses they feel in separating from their families. Their masturbation fantasies eventually mature to spur them on to finding a lover. Not to say that masturbation in itself is immature or that it can't be a lifelong practice. But sexual intimacy is a key force in mate selection driving us beyond ourselves. In early phases of intimacy building, some girls experience deep same-sex friendships occasionally accompanied by sexual experimentation. While for some this marks the beginning of a lesbian sexual orientation, for others it is part of practicing with intensity and sexuality in relationship.

Adolescents practice mating rituals long before they actually have sex. Now, in our technologically brave new world, kids polish their skills via text message, Facebook, Twitter, and instant messaging. Simultaneous conversations help them perfect their dialogue with others. Teens wink, flirt, text, laugh, test, reject, smother, distance, and imitate grown-up love relationships online. Though happy endings—mature and satisfying intimacy—will require much further social, intellectual, and self-development, their feelings are very real at this point.

Precisely because of their lack of experience, adolescent love is intense. Without the defense mechanisms to protect them from possible rejection, young people are especially vulnerable. The first heartbreak may leave them moaning in pain. Parents can be at a loss over their daughter's anguish over the end of an early love. Then they're bewildered by her quick crush on someone else. Tender handling with reflection and observations rather than judgment help a girl organize chaotic feelings about relationships. Say "you are really hurting over him," rather than "well, you weren't going to marry him anyway." Remembering your own first breakup can serve as an empathic guide for the depth of feeling that young people experience. Dismissing their pain as silly or inconsequential only serves to separate parent from daughter, as she feels unsupported and misunderstood in her first relational crisis.

Some families drastically limit their children's sensible exposure to healthy practice situations. In an effort to protect their daughter, they will delay reasonable permission for her to date or restrict her access to normal peer relationships. Once out of their parents' jurisdiction, such kids can wilt when faced with adult sexual challenges. Without preparation in relating and dating guided by thoughtful parental narrative, these college-age kids can be overwhelmed and shrink from healthy relationships or be at sea and drown in the attention of the opposite sex.

Other families have no protective structure around dating. Daughters from these families are often exposed to perilous sexual situations and left without ways to cope and recover when they are hurt. No one really cares. Permissive or negligent family structures do not shield adolescents from the kinds of pain they endure from "failed" efforts at being a couple.[6] Such traumatic scars can permanently handicap future intimacy. Girls in these families are often prematurely sexual, and put themselves in unsafe situations without adequate protection. They seek the affection and attention lacking in their families. They may encounter violence or sexual aggression without feeling that their parents would support or protect their innocence.

Socioeconomic differences in families create different problems for adolescent girls attempting to claim sexual desire for their own. In *Dilemmas of Desire*, Deborah Tolman describes how the socioeconomically disadvantaged urban teenage girls she studied are taught that giving in to sexual desire is tantamount to traveling down the "road to ruination." Their stories particularly reflected fear of sexual violence and a bad reputation. Tolman explains, "Without the message that girls are entitled to sexual desire, self-respect usually translates into a girl's resistance to giving in to a boy's desire; the self in question should not by definition have her own desire."

According to Tolman's study, more economically comfortable suburban girls received mixed messages that "girls can do anything" but that they better not cross an invisible line of doing too much. This tension between directives kept them in a state of anxiety resolved only somewhat by using "romance" as a narrative that protected them from being labeled a slut. Sex became okay if they were in love. Fear of not being regarded as a "good" girl, especially by their mother, kept suburban adolescent females from owning pleasure for its own right. Because of the inherent risks that accompany poverty, and the threat of violence in an urban setting, suburban girls who only faced the possibility of parental disapproval fared better in terms of entitlement to feelings of desire.

And while I am not advocating promiscuity, a girl who feels she must be the one to put on the brakes in every relationship may also not know how to be the engine.[7] We also need to teach our teenage sons to be responsible, to keep sexual relationships congruent with their age and its related emotional-relational possibilities. We need to teach our teenage daughters that their bodies should give them excitement and orgasm, that their sexual desire is healthy and human and good, that they deserve pleasure and priority from a lover when the time is right, and that speaking up for themselves is important for their happiness. We need to teach them to expect respect.

Sexual intercourse that happens before a girl has a strong enough sense of who she is can leave her dependent upon approval from her partner. A young woman must be able to set her own course and decide when she wants to enter the world of intimate pleasure. For a girl without sufficient autonomy and an adequate voice, a sexual relationship can prematurely widen the distance between her and her parents, even if she only believes they condemn her. Because orgasm is an ultimate fusion with another, she may need to break up with her partner just to reestablish her own solidarity of self. But when she is a little older and autonomous enough psychologically, the pleasure of the experience strengthens her bond with her partner, marks her as more independent, and increases their love just as it would in adulthood. According to Scharff, if adolescent love comes at an appropriate time, it can support personal growth just like adult sexuality. "Bodily pleasure can be used in support of an intimate bond."[8]

As a product of positive messages about sexuality, a young woman retains a natural curiosity about nakedness and touch. And when able to bring this natural, unashamed part into adulthood, she approaches sex with playfulness, joy, and love. She explores sensuality without inhibition. She abandons herself to the pleasure of touching and being touched. She is delighted when she sees the mechanism of an erection—her lover's penis changing under her influence. She feels excited when she touches her vulva to find it swollen and slick. Our exuberance about sex or lack thereof is a legacy from our family of origin.

I often ask clients to describe their families and what they learned about sex. My client Natasha, a thirty-two-year-old elementary school teacher, told me, "When I was growing up, sex was not something we talked about. As a child, I guessed it was something bad because my mother never mentioned it. I had to learn from my older, married sister what to do when I started my period. I thought I was dying! So by the time I was kissing and touching boys and they were touching me, there was no way I would have talked about it in my house or anywhere else. I let myself do whatever the boy I was with wanted to do. It felt good to be taken over. Eventually I had an orgasm and my body felt good too." Now, years later, Natasha is quiet in bed about what brings her pleasure.

Deliberately examining the message contained in her mother's silence, Natasha realized many things about her large family. First, her early foray into sexuality came from a hunger for tenderness that was missing in the hustle and bustle of surviving in a home with seven children. As one of the younger siblings, Natasha had been cared for by already-burdened older kids struggling to study, work, or both. She remembered lingering in the bathroom during nail clipping because it was the only time her mother touched her. Natasha came to believe that her mother feared talking about sex because it might make her daughters want to experiment. Instead of preventing early sexuality, the silence only taught Natasha that you couldn't talk about sex. She wouldn't ask her partners to use condoms. And she got into more than a couple of dicey situations that left her feeling used and abused. She decided her desires must be wrong or dangerous. Since her own needs couldn't be trusted, she came to rely on a man to direct the experience. Sex was something that happened to her. Even in marriage, her passivity kept her from comfortably telling her husband about her preferences.

A Long Island transplant in her mid-thirties, Bianca had lovely olive skin and long brown hair. She was a returning client whom I'd seen in her late twenties as she waded through the turbulent waters of the dating scene. After marrying Eric, she had taken a sabbatical from inner therapeutic work. Six years into the marriage now, she had lost her libido. We began reviewing some of her dating relationships and family background to decipher the reasons for her waning sex drive.

"Remember Trent from Utah? The guy who could only get off if he did me from behind?" Bianca began. I confessed I didn't recall him, and she continued: "Well, I didn't date him long, but I really wanted it to work. He was the med student who wouldn't have sex on school nights. I remember admiring his discipline, but now I think he was just uptight and obsessive. Really, he was kind of dead in his soul, but I kept fantasizing about myself as the doctor's wife, so I told myself it would be okay. I know now I would have been unhappy with him.

"Unfortunately, we'd have probably been a match sexually, though; he wasn't very passionate. He wasn't as alive as Eric is. Eric is full of zeal for his work, our children, our friends. He just has tremendous energy about everything, including sex. I don't have anywhere near his get-up-and-go. I'm sure that frustrates him as much as my lack of passion in bed does."

The two things are often related. A shut-down libido results in low energy. Life has no pizzazz. Libido is life energy. Women with libido pulse with electric vigor. Like hot wires, you feel the voltage when standing near them. Some women repress sexuality for fear of losing control; life is safer tame. Tame translated to dead in bed for Bianca. I knew her mother was an alcoholic, and cardinal rules in alcoholic families are: don't talk, don't feel, and don't trust. By this juncture in life, feeling desire felt altogether wrong inside her.

After the death of her grandmother when Bianca was five, her mother had never recovered and started drinking to assuage her grief. Withdrawing from the family, she left Bianca alone to do her homework and deal with the trials of childhood. Bianca eventually took over caring for her younger sister and often started dinner while her mother slept it off on the couch. Over the years, her mother had managed to ruin most holidays with drunken drama, including at Bianca and Eric's wedding. Bianca's mother had argued loudly with Bianca's father during the reception, eventually stumbling, falling down, scraping her knees, and needing to be removed in order to recover, out of sight from the rest of the guests.

"To the rest of the world I was a good kid and good student," Bianca commented, "but my home life was out of control. When Mom was sober she would be overly solicitous—gooey really—and making promises that were always broken. I felt so sorry for my father having a wife that would embarrass him at every turn, so I tried even harder to make him proud of me. He never set any limits with her and on the holidays still expects us to entertain her while she drinks her vodka. I can tell within one word on a phone call whether she's been drinking or not."

Bianca needed affection from her mother, but couldn't trust it when it came. This paradox caused her to shut off her need entirely. Her father had enabled her mother's addiction and never assumed enough responsibility to relieve Bianca of the great pressure she felt for fulfilling the household obligations. In his frustration, he mostly preoccupied himself with his work, leaving Bianca in charge and alone to deal with a frightening situation.

Alcohol also lowers the inhibitions of the drinker, allowing more primitive feelings to emerge. Children of drinkers report many verbal, physical, and sexual boundary injuries at home. Their exposure can run the gamut: harsh or out-of-control physical discipline, precious possessions thrown and broken, too much responsibility (often worse if mother is the alcoholic), possible exposure to the drunk parent's nudity when the latter has passed out, bathroom privacy ignored, financial and economic repercussions, lewd comments, or (though not in Bianca's case) watching a mother groped by a drunk father. Dreadfully, the risk for actual molestation greatly increases in alcoholic families.

The "don't-feel" rule in alcoholic families is a way of minimizing pain in order to survive. Other feelings of bliss, happiness, and sexual desire also get locked into a Pandora's box of repressed memories. "Don't tell" isolates the family from getting help. Children cope in different ways. While one brother becomes an addict, another pours his energy into more constructive endeavors. Yet both may suffer the same emotional shutdown from a traumatic childhood. "Don't trust" can repress our libido. In Bianca's case, she was the family heroine, while her sister played on as the continuing drug addict.

Bianca had a hard time accepting my empathy for her situation. It made her suffering real. She needed to distance herself. "It's like you're talking about someone else's family," she remarked. "I know that what I said sounds bad, but I feel so numb to it. If a friend at work had just told me that story, I'd have said what you just said. But it makes me want to defend my parents and say stuff like, 'It wasn't that bad.' "

Continuing to discuss the past, she added, "But Mom did weird stuff like flirt with my dates. She'd say borderline inappropriate things. Sometimes she'd nudge them and ask if they 'got some.' She'd dress provocatively at school functions. It was like she was in competition with me. So basically, I just kept my dates away from the house and I didn't date much. Flirting felt dirty and reminded me of my mother."

Bianca and I talked about all the stages of sexual growth, and then she continued to reflect further on her mother's direct messages about her sexuality. "My mother wasn't happy about me leaving for college. She'd grown up in the Bronx and left home at sixteen. In fact, it was her guilt, I think, for leaving my grandma with her alcoholic husband that ate my mom up. We've never really discussed it. But she certainly seemed jealous of my opportunity. I felt sorry for her and also felt some guilt wondering how she'd manage without me. When I was a teenager, she was never able to say I looked nice and only seemed to criticize my clothes or my hair. Once when I'd been out with a boy too late, she was furious and slapped my face and told me people would think I was a slut. Mom was always worried about what people would think, except when it came to her drinking. Then she thought it was really a big secret, even though the neighbors and relatives all knew. I remember her weeping about being a bad mother the next day and having to comfort her when actually I was angry and agreed that she was pretty crappy. By no means did I ever sense any magic between her and Dad. Most of the time she just seemed depressed and barely managing to get through life's ordinary chores."

Bianca numbed herself to her first sexual experiences in college with lots of alcohol—a tried-and-true family solution. She confided, "And I didn't get a chance to flirt with the guy because we were already in bed."

Partly because of this background, Bianca's husband's sexual innuendos caused her anxiety. She wasn't comfortable offering a quick comeback. She didn't know what to say. Sex wasn't the only problem. When the seduction process began, she felt as though she was sliding out of control. She trusted Eric and knew the outcome would be safe enough, and yet mentally she couldn't relax. Another part of her had trouble relaxing too.

"When he starts touching me, my right hand stiffens against the mattress. It's like I'm about to be in a car wreck and I'm bracing for impact. It's crazy because I'm starting to have tendonitis in that arm. I notice I have pain there whenever I am under any kind of stress. My left hand can touch and participate, but my right arm is this vigilante. It's like it's hollering, 'Stop!'" As she talked, Bianca looked at her hands. The right one was gripping the chair, while the left gestured freely as she spoke. Her body was saying, "Come here and keep away" all at once.

Our minds and bodies are connected, and if we listen to them, they can give voice to our problems. Talking about what the pain signifies may relieve us of the troubling physical symptoms. Bianca was literally bracing against relaxation. To let her guard down was to invite disaster, as she had discovered in childhood.

Every good expectation had been trashed in some way by her mother's behavior. Sexual pleasure required her to melt into the experience and she tried to split her body in two—one part being sexual and one part being wary.

I also pointed out to Bianca that her low energy—actually a sign of her depression—kept her in her mother's shoes. Except for her college bingeing, she had avoided alcohol. But in a strange effort to maintain a connection with her mother, she couldn't celebrate the joy and kindness she'd found in Eric, worrying instead about becoming a "slut" and confirming her mother's judgment.

A childhood that is disrupted, as in an alcoholic or otherwise chaotic home, may result in disrupted adult sexuality. Parents in these homes simply do not have enough energy left over to nurture children in ways that make intimate relationships natural later in life. Staying erotic for a lifelong relationship demands the ability to risk and let go. When you grow up in a household where "letting go" means dishes start flying or somebody gets drunk, emotional constriction actually makes sense.

Without conscious change, we reduce both the relational and occupational success potential for our own children as well as our current happiness. Fortunately, recalling our history makes us aware of which aspects we are repeating. It gives us a choice about what part from our families we want to replicate. It gives us power over destructive elements that do not serve our adult goals of intimacy, connection, and eroticism. Going forward, we can relate to those we love in a manner of our own shaping rather than imitating familiar patterns or reacting blindly against them. Fortunately, love stands outside of time, and if we can let it in, it can repair the wounds from earlier times. Likewise, to have sexual desire over the long haul, we must become sexually conscious. Allowing ourselves sexual love touches the most primitive parts of our being that crave affection, stroking, tenderness, and excitement.

Help Yourself

1. What were the overt and covert messages about sexuality that you received in childhood?

2. How was touch and affection handled between your parents and between parents and children in your family of origin?

3. Describe your first sexual experience. What do you wish you had known at the time?

4. Does depression accompany your low libido? What wounds from developmental milestones remain unresolved?

· CHAPTER NINE ·

Making Peace with Aversion

Sigrid lived intentionally with a central purpose: being a mother. She was bright and robust, with pale Scandinavian eyes. Her body was a luscious pear, with rounded hips and delicate upper limbs. Her ruddy cheeks on the winter days told me how cold it was outside. Wearing comfortable, flowing knit clothing, she seemed to me a Nordic queen.

Focusing tremendous energy on making the right choices for her children, she swaddled, nursed, and massaged them as infants. Now their nutrition and supplements were guided by holistic medicinal teaching. She'd enrolled them into progressive-thinking Montessori schools. Already, the older kids had seen specialists in reading and family therapy. Rituals and ceremonies marked their family life—all thoughtfully and creatively planned.

Sigrid's feminine energy nurtured her children and had influenced her selection of a husband. She looked for a man who would share her egalitarian beliefs and focus on home. She was deeply committed to living meaningfully and purposefully—except when it came to her sexuality.

Yin and Yang

According to Eastern thought, the individual personality of every man or woman is made of two energies—female and male. While one force may dominate the nature of a person, the ability to access both aspects brings the right strength to any particular task or problem at hand. In theory, feminine energy is about receptivity, intuition, waiting, patience, nurturance, and being inwardly focused. Accordingly, we sometimes observe women using their natural gifts to guide the emotional dynamics of their families. Our respective anatomy and reproductive roles support these ideas: A woman's sexual center is quite hidden between her legs. Her vagina is a receiving space. Her sexuality emanates from her heart, which explains why so many women feel they can't have sex until they feel connected to their partners emotionally.

Masculine energy is active, decisive, logical, production-oriented, hard, and outwardly focused. And in traditional marriages like Sigrid's, husbands focus on the building of hard assets. Sexually, a man is prompted by external stimuli to wish for sexual contact. He sees; he wants. His genitalia proudly wags in front to cross the finish line first. A male body may want sex regardless of the quality of his heart's affection. With action and energy, he directly starts the sexual exchange. If the husband of a low-libido woman gives up initiation, the sexual energy in the marriage is usually abysmally low. Split-off masculine energy in a woman can leave her powerless to get out of a bad marriage. Healthy masculine energy can reenergize her sexually to take concrete steps to rebuild her sex life.

Sigrid's marriage divided roles into breadwinner and bread maker. Sigrid was consciously committed to harmonious relationships. She had unconsciously looked for an androgynous man to marry. Sameness was safe. "Jeremy is a nice man but not a man's man. He's definitely got the well-developed feminine side which I like. At work, he is aggressive enough to make a good living, but at home, he listens to me and wants to talk about our relationship. Ninety-nine percent of the time, he lets me have things my way, because, well, it's his way too. So, getting along is easy. Except that we don't have sex often enough." Sigrid had no problems reaching orgasm. Clearly, she and her husband's relationship functioned smoothly. Together she and I ruled out the common causes of low libido. Showing up early in the marriage, the problems had cemented by the time the children were born and Sigrid immersed herself in their care.

Is It the Kids or Something Else?

"Laurie, my interest evaporated. I never think about sex. When Jeremy asks, I'll give in because of my guilt, but I don't want to. He knows I'm not into it. We end up angrier at each other than before we started making love. But I can't make myself want it. I don't need sex. I'm happy with things the way they are."

"How are you happy when the man you love is not happy?" I confronted this viewpoint. "You say he can tell you're not into it. Do you simply lie there?"

Sigrid sighed. "Probably. While I try not to, I guess I'd rather deaden myself. And it makes me sad for his life; he deserves more than I give him because he is a really good man."

I had come to appreciate Sigrid's sometimes insightful acknowledgment of her own motives. She had acted as though allowing herself to be penetrated fulfilled her feminine calling. She was starting to see how "duty sex" missed the joyful note important to her husband and herself as well. Neither partner used their masculine energy to clear through this muddle of platonic love.

Fidelity's promise is a double-edged sword. Certainly it means keeping away from all others. Sigrid understood and found this aspect easy because she didn't want sex with anyone. But the vow to be faithful deeply commits us also to vibrant sexuality with our spouse. The commitment can be so obvious on a wedding day, with two people so near sexual combustion that onlookers are practically singed by nuptial heat. In fact, weddings are exciting events because of the warmth and sparks they ignite in all of us.

With the chemistry gone, it was almost like Sigrid was an inanimate sex toy for Jeremy to masturbate with. I knew he must have found the arrangement desperate. Pressing on, I asked Sigrid to explain further about her anxious feeling that kept sex an empty, mechanical exchange.

"I felt more sexual when we got married, but I feel a little nervous now. Well, maybe more than just a little nervous. Sort of like how my husband hates to dance. He says he breaks out in a sweat when he thinks about going on the dance floor and just flinging his body all about with everyone watching. I start to get anxious every night thinking Jeremy will want us to do it."

His Stuff Makes Me Nervous

"Jeremy may not be into cars or hunting or sports, but he's definitely into sex. He doesn't even like to settle for a quickie at this point because he says he wants me present." She rolled her eyes. "He wants to know he's making love to me . . . not just to my body. I like the cuddling, but we can never do that because then he gets excited."

"You mean he gets an erection?" I asked evenly.

Blushing, Sigrid hesitated. "See? I don't even know how to talk about sex. It's all so embarrassing. If you must know, when I look at his genitals, I think they're ugly." She shuddered. "Even in the beginning, I didn't really like touching it . . . and blow jobs? Ugh . . . no, never . . . out of the question! I don't think my feelings were as noticeable back then because I still wanted orgasms, and intercourse was fine for that."

As Sigrid explained her anxiety about Jeremy's penis, I realized that she had a sexual aversion to it. At the heart of the matter, Sigrid recoiled at the most intimate maleness of her husband. Her world, with little exception, was a comfortable nest of feminine design. His desire, evidenced by an erection, felt threatening— perhaps threatening to tear her feminine world apart on a primitive level. His penis and testicles abruptly broke her smooth feminine ideal; their existence caused almost a reverse castration anxiety, like they were horrid growths where only a soft mons should be.

Women are invaded at the core of their being during sex. Sigrid in many ways controlled her husband. Her ideas dominated the way they raised their family, spent their time, and spent their money. But in actual sexual intercourse, she was out of control. He was in her. She could not see the need for the masculine in her insular feminine world. While Jeremy was no caveman by her own report, he was still very male.

I checked to see if the root of Sigrid's aversion was actually covering a sexual desire for her same gender. "Do you feel any less anxiety or more desire when you see a naked woman?"

Gathering where I was going with my line of thought, she answered, "I did experiment with a lesbian relationship in college. My best friend and I had a really intense friendship. One night we got drunk and made love and for a short time were sexual. But after the novelty had worn off, I wished we had just remained friends. I know this sounds different than what I've just said about Jeremy, but my feelings of sexual excitement have almost always revolved around men more than women. I like men's smells and bodies and rugged skin; I just don't want to look at them naked. I think women's bodies are beautiful, but mainly because they are familiar. I don't gravitate toward them sexually."

Wading into a more delicate topic, I asked, "What do you not like about looking at your husband's penis?"

Definitively answering, Sigrid said, "It's big and red and erupting. I just feel repulsed when I look at it."

"So his penis offends you. Anything else?" I asked.

"His genitals are just nasty with black hair growing scantily over his sweaty, white, pubic area and purplish balls . . . they're disgusting." She shuddered again.

Hoping for some positive response, I ventured, "Are there any parts of his naked body that you enjoy looking at?"

Taking her time to answer, Sigrid tentatively put forth, "I like his butt. It's smooth, hairless, and white."

More and more I was coming to understand that her low libido was not due to the demands of child rearing. Her desire for control, her repugnance toward her husband's penis, and her deep value of all things feminine and distrust of all things masculine did not begin with the birth of her children.

Sexual aversion translates to disgust and revulsion about the genitals or the sex act itself and often stems from childhood or adult sexual trauma. Scharff clarifies this point: "Massive conflicts barely remembered or long surrendered to the unconscious are projected in condensed form on the body screen of the genitalia."[1] Sigrid had not offered any of these scenarios during our initial information-gathering sessions. She had been more sexually functional during courtship, but perhaps with the advent of childbirth, something from her past began to dominate her sexual feelings and diminish her libido.

In further sessions, I spoke with Sigrid extensively about her childhood and family of origin. When she was growing up, her father had disciplined her brother with a belt. He set nearly impossible standards for the boy, including high academic achievement and military-like cleanliness for his room. For reasons not quite clear to her, Sigrid had avoided her dad's scrutiny and also had been spared the brunt of his cruelty. But her memories included hearing the lashing of her brother's bare bottom in the next room and listening to him weep in the night after he thought everyone was asleep. Forbidden to go to him with comfort or sympathy, Sigrid found herself coping the only way she knew how. She numbed herself and began to wonder if her brother was as bad as her father said. He was sent away to military school at fourteen, and grew into the only type of man her father could respect—mean and hard-hearted.

Sigrid's mother had not intervened to stop the abuse of her son. Instead, she lamented the fact that she didn't know the slightest thing about raising boys and couldn't understand all the trouble he gave them. Weak and ineffectual, she had provided a semblance of family structure by making meals and performing household chores, but warmth and vitality had been missing from the home. Once, Sigrid had begged her to stop Dad from hurting her brother, but her mother had simply shrugged and told her to mind her p's and q's so that she wouldn't get in trouble too. To keep the peace, her mother had sacrificed her son.

To have a penis or to be near the owner of a penis had been dangerous in Sigrid's childhood, and for some time our therapy revolved around repairing the damage to her psyche that had split her off from the masculine. Her sense of safety came from giving to her children all the emotional richness that had been missing in her own family, and indeed it proved a triumph over her upbringing. After considerable work in therapy, we were able to tackle her sexual aversion directly.

Taming Big Red

To tame Sigrid's anxiety about her husband's genitals, we agreed to some steps for progressive desensitization. In a joint session, Jeremy indicated his willingness to try anything I suggested. As a first exercise, Sigrid thought she could touch her husband's genitals through clothing but not if he was erect. As you can imagine, Jeremy found her touch electrifying and his penis immediately responded. Eventually she conceded that feeling his erections through his clothes was unavoidable and not as repulsive as she had thought.

Second, Sigrid allowed him to lie naked next to her with no pressure to exchange touch. After a time she could tolerate seeing his inevitable erections with the understanding that an erection did not demand the release of an orgasm. Eventually, they were able to give and receive massages of their backs, including their buttocks.

After she could tolerate seeing his naked body without feelings of pressure or panic, they were assigned to take showers together. Jeremy was to primarily face away from her while she soaped his body. Touching his penis became possible as long as she did not have to look at the same time.

Unlike most men, Jeremy had no nickname for his penis, so to add some humor and make their experiment seem less clinical, Sigrid named it "Big Red." Some of the seriousness about their sexual exercises began to dissipate. Over time, she could soap Big Red and bring Jeremy to climax.

Although she struggled with it, Sigrid watched a film on manual sexual techniques. She watched acts of touching performed on bigger penises than her husband's and had to calm her rising anxiety. But she did gain ideas on how other men liked to be touched and felt it improved her proficiency. Seeing a series of penises both erect and flaccid reduced her unconscious shuddering defense.

We read all the time about how stress destroys our health,

proving that our bodies and emotions are intractably entwined. As we've begun to see in this book, low sexual desire is often caused by a confluence of issues in our bodies, emotions, and relationships. As a way of dealing with earlier pain or trauma, a burdened mind can channel thoughts or memories into a particular physical symptom or sexual aversion. Sigrid had siphoned her angst from childhood into her husband's penis. In another shift of emotions to the body, her shuddering, we found, corresponded to her intense fear and anguish as she had listened to her brother bear his punishment.

After quite a bit of work on her past, Sigrid began to see the interpersonal issues associated with her aversion. "I felt an old dread seeing those huge penises," she reported upon further reflection on the films. "Huge erection meant huge demand. But I've realized that Jeremy really doesn't expect sex every time he has an erection. We tease a bit now about what Big Red is up to when it happens. Sometimes he says Big Red needs to explode, and if I don't feel like doing him or having sex, Jeremy takes him into the shower. And men are not that complicated. I'm not sure what techniques I was expecting, but much of what I saw in the film, I've already done to Jeremy."

Jeremy had stopped using his erection as the primary signal that he wanted sex and had begun attempting verbal seduction again. And Sigrid's dream life began to reflect healthy themes about arousal, which helped her libido overall and helped repair the tension in her marriage.

Severe sexual anxiety or aversion can take many forms but originates in the psyche because of unresolved issues that then show up in the bedroom. In another instance, one young client could not stand her nipples to be touched in any sexual way.

Therapy revealed that her mother had had breast cancer and a resultant double mastectomy. When her mother's survival was not certain and the threat of death and loss hung over the family, the daughter saw her mother's surgically marred chest with stitches and drains still in place. The intensity of the family's emotional climate juxtaposed with the shock of seeing her mother's mastectomy wounds deeply impacted this early pubescent young girl's sense of her own sexually developing body. For a further example, rape and date rape could easily lead to sexual aversion. Date rape is a common cause of severe phobias about sexual intercourse or sexual contact among my patients. While they may remember the details, the problem is complicated because it involves emotional violation by a trusted person. Women often explain the problems of their shattered sexual self as being caused by low libido rather than by violation. Recovering sexual desire requires the untangling of the body's natural impulse from the mind's hurt.

If early cognitive behavioral therapeutic treatments fail, then deeper psychodynamic therapy, which examines the past and analyzes the unconscious, should be sought to resolve the problems. While Sigrid was able to overcome her sexual aversion with psychotherapy and behavioral instruction, many women with aversions need deeper analysis and sometimes medication. "Highly anxious patients who are undergoing sex therapy should receive anti-anxiety drugs in doses that are high enough to block their panic attacks without interfering with their sexual function," advises sex therapist and renowned sexual leader Helen Singer Kaplan, MD, in *The Sexual Desire Disorders.*

Help Yourself

1. What feminine energy qualities and masculine energy qualities do you value in yourself?

2. Discuss qualities in your partner that attracted you.

3. Do you feel anxious about certain body parts of yourself or of your partner? Is your low desire more diffuse?

4. If you have experienced direct sexual trauma (molestation or rape), contact a therapist to begin the process of healing.

CHAPTER TEN

Easy Prey No More

Growing into our fully sexual selves happens mostly in the mind. Unfortunately, when memories hold trauma, libido can be repressed for a woman's psychic protection. The journey toward a healthy libido after sexual abuse can be difficult and complicated, and recovery from sexual abuse encompasses a lot more than just libido.

Sharon had been molested by her drunk grandfather for two summers during her early puberty while she and her sister were sent to visit. He would regularly take her to the drive-through car wash and rub her genitals, whispering and asking if she liked it when he touched her. She didn't.

In the beginning of her marriage, she pushed these memories far enough down that they didn't interrupt sex with her husband. But things started to change. Soon, when her husband touched her genitals or spoke softly in her ear, it started to feel creepy. In the last fifteen years of her marriage, Sharon had gained thirty-five pounds and thought about the molestation every time they made love. She started to have real headaches whenever her husband wanted sex. Her body screamed about the trauma and she could no longer ignore it. Husbands of victims often know before the woman herself and will relay to me, "I just have an awful feeling that something happened to her." Frustrated, they both wonder why she functioned fine before marriage. Ironically, it's often the very security of marriage that allows memories of childhood molestation to emerge.

"Laurie, this shouldn't bother me. It happened so long ago. I really don't want to talk to anyone about it," she protested in one of our early sessions. She went on to explain, "I hate pity." Unfortunately, many victims of childhood abuse have been encouraged by friends, loved ones, and even professional helpers to simply "let go" of the bad memories and move on with their good life. It is hard to imagine in the beginning how talking about difficult past experiences will bring such a positive change to adult life, including freeing sexual desire by reintegrating the hurt aspects of the personality.

Sharon carried loads of guilt. Intellectually, she knew it wasn't her fault, but she still believed that on some level she was responsible. Sexual abuse is confusing and victims frequently feel riddled with the guilt that belongs to their perpetrator. She worried about the effects on her family. It wasn't that this was a dark secret that would rock them. In fact, her grandfather had molested her sister as well, and their mother came to know about it. Sharon didn't want to make her mother feel worse.

"My sister actually told my mom that she was being molested.

Then my mom asked me if Grandfather was touching me and I remember nodding. That's the only time I admitted it to anyone. Mom seemed upset and didn't really talk to me about it, but he stopped after that conversation. I don't think we were ever left alone with him again. I've become suspicious that my mom might have been molested too," Sharon said.

When a child or adolescent tells an adult that she is being sexually abused, the best outcome for her psychological well-being and sexual self is to be believed. Then the adult takes quick action and stops the abuser. Next, the child should be told it is not her fault and helped to understand that the perpetrator was wrong and sick and the experience should be thoroughly talked about. If the abuser was a person of trust in the child's life, then more help is necessary to rebuild a life where people can be seen as trustworthy. While the child still has to cope with the violation of her body and sexuality, she is reassured that people will protect her and that the world can still be a good place.

In Sharon's case, her mother did believe her and did take action. Unfortunately, the essential debriefing about the specifics of the abuse and her pain over it did not happen. She was left to make sense of it on her own. The legacy of sexual abuse and incest is often denial. Sharon's mother probably was molested and, in order to preserve a semblance of relationship with her parents, denied the horrendous fact of incest. She blithely sent her daughters to their home over the summer and holidays. Vulnerable and alone over vacation, the sisters heard one message from their mother—that their grandfather was a good, loving, and religious man—but lived the opposite reality, that he was a perverted, sexually abusing, and selfish alcoholic.

Sharon worried that if she brought up the sexual problems

she had now, her mother would feel guilty about the past abuse and her sister might be affected too. I asked her what her sister's sex life was like. She confided, "You know, she seems fine. I know she talks easily about sex and she always wants to go into Victoria's Secret to buy sexy things when we're at the mall. She's married now and sex seems a nice part of their life. She seems to look forward to date nights and being alone with her husband. Every once in a while she'll make a sexual joke." I hoped that Sharon's sister had told their mother immediately after her own experience of abuse and that her presumed good sexual adjustment was genuine. As Sharon's therapist, I also knew that to bring the subject up for the family could unleash the huge rage she felt at her mother for endangering her in the first place.

The Vulnerable Girl

It has been estimated that 15 to 25 percent of children are sexually abused by the time they are eighteen years old, and the rates for girls may be closer to 40 percent.[1] In no way, however, do I underestimate the suffering of boy victims. As a world, we have watched in horror and shock as reports of sexual abuse have emerged from boys (and girls) at revered religious and academic institutions. Sexual abuse ranges from incestuous innuendo, inappropriate touching, naked exposure, sexual stimulation, oral sex, to full penetration and forceful rape. How early the abuse begins, how long it lasts, the violence accompanying it, and the closeness of the victim's relationship to the abuser determine the degree of psychic destruction.[2] Alcoholism in the home means that a child is three times more likely to be victimized sexually.[3] A child doesn't tell anyone who could help her because to do so often endangers herself, her mother, her mother's relationship, her siblings, and her economic survival. Most children do not report the abuse—ever. When children do tell, the odds of their making up the incident are less than 1 percent. Despite that statistic, many parents and caregivers refuse to believe a child's reports of abuse and, tragically, if the child is not believed, the damage sustained is much greater. The child begins to question reality itself if her experience is contradicted by those she loves and trusts. If no rescue comes from somebody dependable, the injury is compounded. First, there is the intimate betrayal and then there is abandonment.

Early incest can cause terrible disorganization in a girl's maturing personality and her later sexual functioning. When molestation happens at the height of a young girl's physical development, she often believes that her budding sexuality and beauty were the enticement. Victims feel guilty for their supposed seductiveness, their acceptance of gifts in exchange for keeping the secret, their reluctance to report the abuse, and the false belief that they could have stopped it despite being young, dependent, and powerless. And if their body's natural response to inappropriate stimulation included their own sexual arousal, their guilt is multiplied. Low libido is not evidence of molestation, but unrecovered trauma always compromises sexuality.

Molestation often causes self-hatred. A child is injured directly through the molestation and indirectly by the lack of action to protect her. Those overwhelming feelings of degradation and fears that she deserved it are stowed away to be handled at a later time. The child feels she is bad. Until this damage is processed and worked through as an adult, it will negatively affect her self-image and her ability to have loving sexual relationships. While escape may be impossible during the incidents of molestation themselves, disconnecting from and hating your body is the closest thing possible to leaving the crime scene. Dissociation between the nighttime, abused, terrified child and the daytime, ignorant, functioning schoolgirl is a common way to survive long-lasting childhood molestation.

Abuse survivors sometimes try to rid the demons of unwanted sexual relations through promiscuity. Wendy Maltz, author of *The Sexual Healing Journey*, writes, "Offenders treat victims as sexual objects . . . with no respect or regard for the victim's humanity or rights." As a result, victims can see sex as a commodity or use it to please others instead of as a gift shared between two people who respect and care about each other. They give their sex to as many partners as there are who want it, repeatedly demonstrating that their sexuality is cheap and meaningless, which in turn affirms the message of the perpetrator. Promiscuous reenactment is not pleasurable or satisfying sex but often shame-filled, robotic, and addictive. Oftentimes the violent abuse is reenacted by repeated relationships with abusive men and, for some, sadomasochistic sex acts.

Surviving in adulthood, in many cases, means shutting down libido and sexual contact. Sexual arousal can trigger an array of symptoms characteristic of post-traumatic stress disorder: flashbacks, nightmares, panic attacks, severe anxiety, zoning out, and obsessions about the abuse. Physical symptoms with unexplained origins can be another signal of childhood abuse. Sexual pain problems are sometimes the manifestation of previous molestation.

Once the triggers for these overwhelming experiences are understood, it makes sense to want to avoid them. But this doesn't help a marriage. To restore marital intimacy, the goal in therapy is full integration of the memories and healing from the distorted childhood relationships.

I wasn't surprised that Sharon's sister's libido seemed stronger than her own. Whistle-blowers often survive sexual abuse better than secret keepers. Somehow, whistle-blowers are able to value themselves above the family's false values of peacekeeping or keeping up appearances. Remaining silent to protect the family from disruption or shame or potential further abuse is usually a worthless sacrifice anyway. There usually have already been other casualties as well. Many times, survivors of sexual abuse within the family tell me of sisters, brothers, cousins, and parents who have been molested, sometimes by the same person. The abuser is not a respecter of age or gender and does not spontaneously rehabilitate. Sexual molestation, like rape and date rape, is an act of power and violence, injecting the bad, hateful, and guilty parts of the offender into the victim.

Sharon needed to tell her husband and talk about her experience with her family. Telling the story to others breaks the shame of the silence and opens the secret that ties a woman to her perpetrator. Most sexual traumas cannot be processed with the people involved and sometimes it's not safe—psychically or even physically—to attempt to do so. A person depraved enough to sexually molest a child usually does not take responsibility for his or her actions.

Sharon's husband had no idea about the past abuse and was suffering its consequences in his heart and in their marriage. From what I gathered, he was the type of man who loved her through thick and thin, literally and figuratively. I believed he would be able to assist in her sexual healing once he knew what was behind her rejection.

Sharon did talk to her husband and told me what happened the next time we met. "You were right, Laurie. He sat in silence through my whole spiel. Then he put his arms around me and started to cry. And you know it's hard for me to be held. He had thought I just didn't love him. He was so relieved and he was so sad for me that he just kept saying over and over again how it wasn't my fault. It was like he cried when I should have been crying."

His affirmations of her innocence were a balm to her self-recriminations. The marriage started to mend and sexual contact was slowly broached. Sharon was ready to bring her husband in for a joint session. I instructed him to stop making love if he sensed her stiffening or withdrawing. We both gave her permission to stop a sexual encounter if memories surfaced. Her ability to receive touch increased as she learned how quickly he'd release her and give her the freedom to rest or roll away. Together, they broke her association of holding with restriction and and violation.

After months of therapy, Sharon began to exercise and take some pride in her appearance again. With agonizing poignancy she said, "I've hated my body. My breasts and genitals seemed like a liability. I think my weight helped turn me into a blob that was anything but sexual because deep down inside, there was a developing child who was terrified. I was protecting her."

Once adequate healing of the sexual abuse has reached a stage where concrete sexual intervention is appropriate, sex therapy can provide a tailored pathway to reduce the anxiety of sexual contact and increase the pleasure of bodily sharing. When a memory is triggered and brought into consciousness, a woman can request a neutral touch while she reorients herself to the present moment. Some women like to be cuddled and held. Others like to lie separately and have their back stroked. Some prefer intense eye contact and soft talking to reassure themselves that they are in the here and now, and not back with their perpetrator. To keep anxiety low while regaining sexual expression, sexual-trauma healing expert Maltz recommends breaking sexual acts into smaller more tolerable steps. For example, "rubbing egg white between the fingers as a step toward feeling comfortable with vaginal secretions or semen; holding the little fingers together as a step toward holding hands; giving and receiving butterfly kisses as a step toward kissing with lips; having a squirt gun fight in the shower as a step toward feeling comfortable with a male partner's ejaculation."[4] Additionally, Maltz suggests that a survivor find one place on her partner's body that feels safe, perhaps laying her head on their chest and listening to their heartbeat, for times when panic or flashbacks interrupt the sexual experience.

Sins of the Father

Elinor, an articulate, intelligent teacher, was nearly sixty when she came for treatment and revealed the sexual molestation she had experienced during childhood. She had *never* married and had very little sexual contact throughout her life. Constant depression had plagued her for as long as she could remember. Recently, she started to have panic attacks.

"It's time to deal with all this stuff," she explained during our initial interview when I asked why she'd come to therapy now.

"My parents are long dead and there is no one who would care. But I realize I've probably missed out on happiness and certainly on marriage or partnership. Now there is a woman who has told me she would like to be more than friends. I know she would want sexual contact if we were to spend more time together. I don't exactly want sex, but I do think this might be a relationship worth having."

Elinor blandly told a horrific story of her innocence stolen and her trust in people permanently scarred. Her father had molested her from age four through high school, eventually including full intercourse. As she spoke about the past, Elinor revealed her suspicion that her mother, a weak and dependent woman, had known but let it continue. Many times victims of sadistic or long-term abuse remember they were molested but specific memories are locked away. And with those details, the spontaneity and joy of their personality are also lost.

Eventually she said, "When I was little, my father was scary. Fortunately, he wasn't around much. He'd be angry at my mother, brother, or me for nearly any reason. I didn't really know that what he did to me was wrong because it did feel good and it was the only time I can remember my father being tender with me. In the beginning, he only touched me. It was such a delightful sensation, I let "our time" outweigh the repulsion I felt for him during his outrages. Eventually he started to have me touch him as well. Then he pressed me for oral sex and I remember gagging. I couldn't have been more than nine and I started to dread his nighttime visits. After a time I felt guilty about my mother—like I was stealing her partner. I would lie still and hope he wouldn't think I was awake, but nothing stopped him. Then I'd lie still during the whole encounter. In fact, sometimes I kept my eyes shut the whole time. You'd think that would've stopped him, but it didn't. I would feel dirty when I'd realize that I was aroused. By the time I was a teenager and my friends were all giddy about sex, I was done with the whole thing. I never wanted to have sex again if I could help it. It's amazing that I didn't get pregnant, but my father would pull out and spew all over my stomach or sheets or pajamas. I have anxiety now if I spill water on my pajamas when I'm brushing my teeth or sipping tea while I read in bed. He'd call me his 'sexy girl,' and since I had been so responsive in the beginning, I believed that I probably had seduced him."

The economic dependency of women from her mother's generation might have made leaving the marriage more difficult, but Elinor had suffered an enormous penalty for her mother's lack of courage. She had grown up not trusting other women enough to form friendships with girls in college or early adulthood. Only after years of professional association had Elinor found women friends at the school where she taught.

Ever the good girl, until our appointment she had never told anyone about the abuse directly—though one of her friends suspected as much by her reactions to discussions about sex. The abuse had stopped when Elinor had written a detailed and lurid story for her high school English class. Concerned that her story indicated that Elinor was promiscuous, her teacher called her parents. There was never a discussion or reprimand, but her father's late-night visits stopped. Today, Elinor mused, "Perhaps my father got nervous over potential exposure. I remember both parents avoided looking at me. I felt a mix of power and blame. I realized my father was afraid of me, but their silence seemed to accuse *me* of the inappropriate behavior."

Not only does prolonged trauma damage a woman's sexuality

catastrophically, it profoundly cripples the core of the self. Frequently, as was the case with Elinor, a person's ability to connect with others is deeply compromised and the ability to feel anything is muted by constant depression. She required long therapy to heal the split between the abused child part and the adult self who wanted to move on with life. Speaking of the treatment necessary for dissociation, psychoanalysts Jody Messler Davies, Ph.D., and Mary Gail Frawley, Ph.D., write: "[it] is in fact undertaking two patients: an adult who struggles to succeed, relate, gain success, and ultimately *to forget* and a child who as treatment progresses, strives *to remember* and to find a voice with which to scream out her outrage at the world" (emphasis added).[5] Reconciling these two aspects of a victim requires full memory recall of the trauma within the therapeutic relationship that symbolically holds the rage and shame of the wounded child. The world of interpersonal relationships has to be straightened out during the processing of memories. The loss of a happy childhood must be mourned over time with aching grief.

First, the core of the woman must be reintegrated. While some clients are frustrated by a lack of specific memories, with patience, the mind will reveal the painful recollections. Sometimes, I'm asked if hypnosis would assist in gaining access to the forgotten but suspected history. Hypnosis might strip away the defenses of the victimized child part before she is ready. This just leaves her feeling violated again. Many hypnotists, who are not full psychotherapists, are not trained to manage the emotional devastation that can be wrought when oblique hunches become real memories for the first time.

Sex therapy with specific goals of repairing the sexual self might be premature for dissociated survivors. However, the sexual needs of the spouse or life partner during her therapy have to be considered as well. As far as possible, I believe viable marital relationships or life partnerships must be supported in order to heal the attachment problems that result from the betrayal of trust the abused woman felt toward caretaking figures in childhood. If the adult part of the woman is able to continue with some sexual contact, it is important to do so in order to nourish the marriage. If this proves impossible, the spouse, who is often already sexually deprived, must be brought into the therapy to manage their disappointment and discouragement, and to develop a team mentality toward the goals of the treatment.

Much later and with supreme courage, Elinor entered her first intimate relationship in life with a kind woman about her own age. Her partner's patience and desire for whole body contact allowed Elinor to warm up slowly to sexual arousal. Eventually, Elinor found that contact with a woman's soft body and skin helped lessen the aversion she believed she would have felt over a man's roughly textured body. Often, her partner would simply hold her against her chest while Elinor listened to her heartbeat.

Sexual abuse is a horrendous reality that damages the sexuality of a woman—her arousal, her climax, her body image, her later intimate relationships, even her essence. Therapeutic healing can restore the many losses of the sexual exploitation and bring back the natural life force of desire. When all the lost parts of the damaged child are healed, a woman can have passionate freedom in her adult sexual relationship.

Help Yourself

1. What were the boundaries in your family of origin around privacy, affection, nudity?

2. What was considered "family talk"—information to be kept inside the family—and what information was shareable with friends and relatives? Do you feel comfortable now with these boundaries?

3. Who was family to you as a small child? Who were your caretakers?

4. Do you have any specific memories of sexual inappropriateness or abuse? (Consult with a therapist if the answer is yes.)

CHAPTER ELEVEN

Too Sad for Sex

Depression and anxiety both cause women to feel blasé about having a sexual encounter. Without the playfulness and lightheartedness that make sex fun, depressed women often see nothing to look forward to in the experience, and the low self-worth that often accompanies depression stops a woman from communicating her pleasure. Anxiety, on the other hand, robs a woman of the relaxation in body and mind that she needs to become aroused. It's a vicious circle: mood disorders lower libido and low libido contributes to mood disorders.

Janet, thirty-five, a quiet, thin woman married for seven years, had struggled with mild depression all her life. She hardly allowed herself to sit on my couch or to take a deep breath of air in my office. Her muted, olive, solid black, or generic brown clothes all looked the same to me. Her quiet, reserved manner was probably mistaken for shyness by her colleagues. She told me, "I'm always insecure; it's like I don't deserve my husband or any good things that happen. When I accomplish something, I think it's a fluke. I just can't enjoy my life, so I'm always kind of miserable." Mild depression is a dull, long-standing condition (at least two years), different from grief's sharp pain over the death of a loved one and not as obvious to the outside observer as more severe depression. You feel hopeless, irritable, experience changes in sleep patterns, changes in appetite, an inability to concentrate, and lose interest in regular activities—including sex. Even women who are productive at work and live seemingly full lives can have their world marred by not being able to feel contentment. Many times they don't even know why they are depressed. There is no internal calm to make them believe tomorrow will be better, soothe them during upsets, or assure them that they are still a good person.

To a woman suffering from depression, relational problems may feel like the end of the world because she can't believe that her partner can be angry at her and still love her. Janet felt anxious about the growing coolness between her and her husband, Gary, even though she caused much of it with her emotional and sexual rejection. "I know I'm the one who's pulling away. I love my husband and I don't want to lose him. I never think about sex and I know that's wrong. I remember feeling sexy and happy, but it seems like a distant dream. And I'm too tired for anything, anyway."

When she was falling in love, Janet's depression seemed to disappear. She had felt sexually alive and daring. Briefly into the marriage, though, the cloud of despondent feelings crept over her again. She had withdrawn into her work and found little time for the things they had been enjoying together, like biking and cooking. She lost interest in sex and felt inhibited.

Gary encouraged her to go for therapy, not only so their sex life would improve, but because he loved her and wanted her to feel happy. Invited to one session, he confided, "She came from a tough background and doesn't realize how many people respect her and like her. She rarely lets me tell her I love her and I do love her a lot."

What to Do About It

Treating depression means getting to the root of loss and rejection. The therapeutic relationship can help someone repair the damage from earlier times that might have impaired current relationships. Often therapy alone can cure depression.

Sometimes, though, medications are used along with the talking cure. Selective serotonin reuptake inhibitors (SSRIs) are a class of antidepressants that help prolong the circulation of your own serotonin in your body. Often these medications—Prozac (fluoxetine), Celexa (citalopram), Luvox (fluvoxamine), Zoloft (sertraline), Paxil (paroxetine), and Lexapro (escitalopram)—are an excellent choice. They alleviate both depressed and anxious feelings all in one pill. Sometimes, sexuality and desire can finally reemerge when the depression lifts. These drugs, however, are infamous for causing secondary sexual problems of low libido and difficulty with orgasm.[1]

Sometimes, clients are already on medication when they come to see me. And sometimes, that medication might be causing the low libido. But changing a medication can be problematic. Stopping a medication to help with sexual desire may not be right for a woman's mental health. I try to work with clients to find every other issue that might be causing low desire before sending them back to a psychiatrist for a medication reevaluation. No one should make an independent decision to go off an existing medication without being under the careful supervision of their doctor.

Janet had been put on an SSRI when she was in her twenties and had been treated by therapy that emphasized positive thinking. It hadn't helped much. Both Janet and Gary wanted to understand why the meds were interfering with her desire and ability to climax now but had not affected her during their dating years. A new love relationship is so exciting and so erotically charged that past difficulties and inhibitions are overcome. Even hormonal deficits can be conquered in both men and women when they experience expansive sexual feelings while falling in love. When a relationship becomes real, with conflicts and genuine needs, some of the high wears off and we have to work through physical or psychological stumbling blocks.

Janet's individual therapy centered around her depression for a long time. When she came to see me, we talked about how her need for affection and touch went underground after she got married. At first, it just wasn't important to her. But when a person denies physical love, there are often deep psychological roots strangling their natural longing for affection and love. Janet had been rejected and neglected as a child. Her mother was very young and hadn't wanted a child. Her father wasn't in the picture. Janet would sleep wherever her mother was partying for the night. Once, the school principal called her mom to say that unless Janet came to school with a bath and clean clothes, he'd call social services.

Janet managed the deep sadness she felt by being apathetic about her intimate life with her husband. Like many depressed people, she could not let others love her—love that would heal the depression. To someone suffering from depression, trusting others to meet your needs is foolish and leaves you dangerously vulnerable. Intellectually, she could see how much her husband loved her, especially with his patience over her sexual rejection. But physical desire just seemed too risky. So she rejected him before he could reject her by turning off her desire.

As we progressed, she began to meet her husband's sexual needs. But she couldn't yet recognize her own. After a year of therapy, she started to notice that even though she felt vulnerable during sex, she felt more secure afterward. Risking, not avoiding, made her feel better. Eventually, she felt safe enough to make suggestions and to respond with a moan or sigh when she felt good. Initiation was the hardest thing to try but Gary was pleased that Janet could be responsive and remained patient.

For a woman on SSRIs, I highly recommend the use of a vibrator to counter the deadening effects of the medication. Vibrators aren't just sex toys but necessary tools so she doesn't get too discouraged. They can build arousal quickly and help a woman handicapped by medication reach climax without worrying that she's "taking forever." Orgasm can break through depression's gloom with that one ecstatic moment and bring hope of good things about life and her body.

Other Types of Medication
Sex Effects

For depression without anxiety, some physicians prefer dopamine-enhancing medications like Wellbutrin because they lack the frequent sexual side effects—low libido and slow orgasm—of the SSRI drugs. Other medications or drug combinations can be used to stop anxiety or panic attacks. Since the most urgent issue is alleviating the mood disorder, sometimes patients are not told about the sexual-debilitating consequences or given a choice of medications.

For the best quality of life, make sure to work with your psychiatrist to find solutions for the sexual side effects of any medication. Under his/her careful supervision, some medications for depression or anxiety may allow for a drug "holiday" or dose reductions for brief "honeymoon" periods that restore more bodily desire. Testosterone also might be used to increase desire with the added benefit of helping reduce depression. Some women on SSRIs are prescribed sildenafil citrate (Viagra or a Viagra cream applied to the clitoris) to try to counter the dampening effects of the SSRI when arousal doesn't result in climax. Viagra does not produce desire in women (or men for that matter) but can relax the arteries in the clitoris to allow better swelling and its normal mini-erection. Sensitivity from the engorgement may produce more pleasure, making orgasm easier.

Other common libido-lowering medications are certain blood pressure medications, sedatives, and antianxiety medications. Conditions and diseases, and their complications and treatments, can limit sexual desire and response: alcoholism, prescription drug addiction, menopause, low thyroid, diabetes, coronary heart disease, peripheral artery disease, multiple sclerosis, and cancer. Sex therapy can analyze which sexual side effects are caused by the disease and which might be caused by more practical problems like lack of stimulation, lack of communication, or lack of relational connection. Tell your physician everything, especially about feelings of low sexual desire, in order to accurately present your health profile and get help for medically correctable libido problems.

Postpartum Depression

Postpartum depression is driven by the changing hormones of pregnancy. A history of depression makes a woman susceptible, but some women experience mood disorders for the first time post-partum. Despite societal expectations, most women have mixed feelings about the process of becoming a mother that are not always adoring, happy, and excited—and they're normal, healthy feelings. We give up tremendous amounts of autonomy to care for infants and small children and—especially while carrying the child and during infancy—always more than their fathers give up. While many women enjoy pregnancy, some feel as if their uteruses are hosting an alien being. They feel taken over by the new life they're creating. Our bodies are stretched out of shape. When we nurse, our lives are not our own and we might feel more like a food source than a caregiver. Then we must navigate our way through a new parenting relationship with our husband or partner. The limited maternity leave granted in American business means that as soon as we bond with our baby, we have to let go in order to return to work. With such increased responsibility and reduced time, energy, and space, we feel claustrophobic. Sexual intimacy can feel distressingly invasive and take a higher emotional toll than at other life stages. To preserve autonomy, distancing sexually can be one of the only decisions a new mother feels is in her control.

All of these changes make most postpartum women feel blue even if they're not suffering from depression. Adding sexual pressure into the mix is hardly a libido stimulant.

But sometimes, the normal blues turn black.

Annie, overwhelmed by her toddler and nursing infant, came to see me a few months after the birth of her second child. She had been depressed as a teenager. She'd been on and off antidepressants during her marriage, and her sex drive was low. Suffering more than just the typical postpartum blues, Annie stopped holding her baby. She was terrified of contaminating him with household dirt and her own germs. Her hands had become raw from washing them. Showering to get ready to nurse was impractical and her nipples had started to hurt. Sex seemed like a mess of dangerous bodily fluids. Yet her infant son's emotional welfare and future capacity for intimacy depended on Annie's feeling connected and being able to hold and care for him. Annie needed to feel close with the baby in order to bond. This was a crisis.

Annie knew what she was experiencing wasn't normal. She had nursed her first child and had not had postpartum depression with that baby. Her husband and her relatives were starting to worry about her state of mind. Luckily, she had no fears of actively hurting the baby or herself.

I asked Annie to think about psychological ways she might feel too bad or dirty to touch her son. "I'm wishing I could just walk out of the house and that makes me a bad mother. With our daughter, Millie, I was nervous about mothering, of course. But, I really wanted children, so I was happy being pregnant and the birth was easy. I felt sick the whole time with Mathias and then I had to have a cesarean because he had gotten so fat. I was gestationally diabetic and I guess I poisoned him with all the sugar I ate."

I assured her that she hadn't poisoned her baby. Gestational diabetes can be hard on a woman's body. It's dangerous to the mother because the baby, not diabetic, puts on weight from the extra sugar in her bloodstream, making delivery harder. Certainly a more difficult pregnancy and delivery can affect our maternal adjustment.

What else was going on with Annie? "I grew up with my sisters and my mom. My brother went to live with my father when he was eight and I was ten. Mom couldn't handle him because he was ADHD [attention-deficit/hyperactive disorder] and always had tantrums. My dad blamed my mom for the divorce and for the way Owen behaved. I missed my brother but was relieved how peaceful things were at home after he left. My mom always felt guilty about sending him away and they've never been close since."

Unconsciously, Annie had gotten the message that raising a boy meant doing the wrong thing and then having to reject him after you had failed. Guilt and blame were main ingredients in her family of origin's stew of love, rejection, marriage, mothers, fathers, and sons. I wondered if Annie was prematurely washing her hands of the guilt she felt from loving her son. The real poison she was afraid of was the feminine and masculine mix.

Relieved at this revelation, she answered, "I think I do feel a huge worry that I just won't do it right. I have no idea what to expect from Mathias and I'm afraid Millie will be left out. But maybe I can learn."

Straightening out the parenting relationship meant we could start thinking about the marital and sexual relationship between her and her husband. "Mike's proved to be a trooper these last few weeks. He took time off work and hasn't complained about how crazy I've seemed. But when we tried to have sex, it hurt. I'm afraid my vagina has been damaged or something. Then my breasts started leaking all over us and I just had to get up and get to the shower." Emotionally, sex seemed like overload given the concerns she was juggling.

Most postpartum women feel a little nervous about their first sexual intercourse after a vaginal birth. Birth and/or episiotomy can traumatize the nerves and tissues of the vagina, resulting in tenderness.

Prolactin, the nursing hormone necessary for milk production, can also make the vaginal tissue thinner and drier even for women who gave birth through cesarean delivery. It also naturally lowers desire. After a woman has stopped breast-feeding, prolactin can stay in her system for months.

There is a definite physical reason for low-libido postpartum. Orgasms from clitoral stimulation during those weeks will bring good blood flow to the area to aid healing. Women should gently stretch their own vaginas in the shower for two weeks before intercourse using a lubricant in order to work through any pain due to the tears of childbirth or episiotomy. Put your fingers in your vagina and gently push down toward the perineum. Massaging this tissue helps get you ready for intercourse. I recommend that all new mothers ask their physicians about the appropriateness of vaginal estrogen for a couple of weeks before having sex to make it less painful.

Leaking breast milk is also normal. Women who are squeamish about it can wear a bra to bed or have a towel handy.

Annie and I discussed developmental issues for boys and their need to be connected to their mothers. We talked through the difficulties in her family of origin and how her brother had been both a victim and a stressor. I communicated with her gynecologist and we arranged an additional appointment for her to be reassured about her post-partum body.

The sexual relationship has to have enough flexibility to sustain occasional rejections. If it becomes a pattern, it can lead to marital unhappiness, but ironically, the path to yes has to come through the right to say no. In addition to saying no to sex once in a while, we have to guard our free time and energy during these child-rearing years. We need to say no to family and friends' requests for too many commitments and no to an inequitable division of household work and child care.

Help Yourself

1. Discuss the times in your life that you have most struggled with depression or anxiety.

2. If you ever used medication to mitigate the mood symptoms, did you experience sexual side effects?

3. If you have children, when do you feel you really became a mother? Did your self-image or body-image change with pregnancy?

4. What repercussions did you feel sexually after motherhood?

CHAPTER TWELVE

Don't Touch My Stomach

No matter how lean, voluptuous, gorgeous, or young a woman is, rarely do I have a conversation with one who's at peace with her body. Thankfully, being in the throes of passion can erase some of these self-critical feelings. But in many low-libido women, a poor body image remains a central culprit that inhibits freedom in the bedroom. For these women, the rules tend to be lights out, under the covers, and perhaps clothes on to hide the parts that jiggle or the parts that don't. One client won't be on top because her husband will be able to see her dimply thighs; another won't let her boyfriend do her from behind because she thinks her bottom is too big. Athletically fit women tell me their breasts are too small, so they won't readily undress in front of their lovers, and dazzling, curvy women tell me their breasts are too big, so they wear shirts in bed.

Barry McCarthy, author of *Rekindling Desire,* sums up the problem this way: "Nothing makes you feel less sexual than feeling self-conscious." Rather than risk being judged unattractive and perhaps rejected, sometimes women would rather draw the curtain on their nakedness and put away their libido.

My immigrant grandmother probably never saw any movies or glossy magazines before she married. She would have compared herself only with other actual women in her immediate neighborhood. She lived at a time when women were valued for attractiveness, certainly, but also for integrity, common sense, warmth, intelligence, humor, nurturance, and diligence. Now, in the media age, women can't help but compare themselves to a tiny fraction of women worldwide who are considered the most attractive.

With a few exceptions, the actresses who play romantic leads have only a portion of their career to play that part before they are cast as mothers and older female characters. Male actors seem to enjoy the "romantic lead" status for more years. Advertisements show unnaturally thin and beautiful women whose flaws and wrinkles have been airbrushed or Botoxed away. It's perfection. It's false. Industry has one goal: to make money. It's such a slick game, we hardly realize we're being conned. "The advertisers who make women's mass culture possible depend on making women feel bad enough about their faces and bodies to spend more money on worthless or pain-inducing products than they would if they felt innately beautiful," asserts Naomi Wolf in *The Beauty Myth.*

This age of the Internet makes things even worse. It's threatening and true that a certain percentage of men have their libido seared by the pornographic images of unattainable body types and eventually learn to prefer impersonal sex to sensual lovemaking with a real female partner. Facebook and other social networking sites offer a perpetual school reunion, making formerly young, juicy lovers easily accessible and offering a partial, best-foot-forward glimpse at their lives now.

Some men and women do seem to be on a quest for perfection in a partner. A young man in therapy recently told me, "It's like the proverbial hunt for a needle in the haystack, which now seems utterly possible using the Internet. Reasonably attractive women who are good conversationalists and would be the catch of the evening at a live cocktail party are passed over in the online search for someone with equal characteristics but ever more attractive." I can only presume that men like my client are seeking Cinderella in an attempt to ensure future attractiveness, desire, and loads of sex.

What Really Attracts

Feeling attractive and being attracted to your partner are such basic necessities for sexual chemistry that it would be unthinkable to live without them. Some couples, though, who do marry for more practical partnership reasons, can use hot sex to release the love hormone oxytocin and deepen their feelings of physical connection. I would argue that what's required for instant attraction is a more complicated formula than the purely biological one of finding the "good breeder"—the hourglass-shaped woman or the V-shaped, strong, protector male.

Our unconscious has an agenda when it comes to attraction. At the beginning of a romance, we are blissfully unaware of our own conflicting feelings about connection. Our partner is handsome (to us); we are beautiful (to him); all is well. Attraction is made up in part by our own projection. We see what we want to see. Romance wears rose-colored glasses.

Partly, in an effort to find a suitable attachment, our unconscious guards us from some of the less desirable aspects of our future lover until we are committed. We deny the shadow side of our partner that later causes us to repeat the adage "beauty is only skin deep."

We also deny any ambivalence about being committed to someone. Wanting what we don't have yet (connection or commitment) allows us to ignore what we also need and want (autonomy and independence). After our commitment we realize our needs for separateness and, unconsciously, our partner's attractiveness can be downgraded. In an effort to detach, we start to focus on their imperfections—his nose is too big, her stomach not as firm, his hair thinner than we saw before, the annoying way she picks her teeth, his pedantic explanations, etc. Losing our feelings of attraction is a perfect foil to claustrophobic closeness.

The longer the commitment, the greater the potential loss and the more power we hand over to our lover to reject us. Our increasing vulnerability demands a defense. Frequently, in the course of therapy I will hear both men and women arriving at more vulnerable relational stages and almost rewriting history to say, "I think maybe I was never attracted to my partner in the first place." Lack of attraction is so subjective—it's inarguable. We believe attraction to be essential to a sexual partnership. We don't realize that our feelings of attraction were in large part due to our investment of time, energy, and a temporary blind eye. Since sex is so intimate and so fragile, it becomes the marital area most at risk of disruption.

Psychological issues can suddenly appear and strain libido. Perhaps our partner's body metamorphoses into our parent of the opposite sex and brings about frightening associations. For instance, perhaps a man chooses a woman who is petite, slim, small-chested, and independent. Then, when she's pregnant, her breasts grow heavy and her emotional state is temporarily a more dependent one. Rather than being stimulated by the culture's penchant for big boobs, this man may begin to see his mother's smothering breasts and body, which symbolized, to him, her clinging, suffocating personality. Suddenly he is repulsed by his young wife. Or a man gains a paunch and, in her head, a woman hears her domineering, narcissistic father's voice denigrating men who don't keep fit; she now finds her partner too soft to feel continued desire. Or a partner's aging can bring your own mortality into closer range, and somehow finding a younger model staves off the scary mirror. Attraction, at all times in a relationship, is filtered through psychological issues. It's never quite an objective judgment.

Working through the loss of physical attraction requires dealing with the psychological difficulties of commitment. First, we must learn not to withdraw because of our own fears of absorption as we grow closer in the relationship. We must accept that our partner could not be everything we wanted them to be but is a real human being with flaws and failings and usually good enough to be a satisfying sexual and emotional partner. We must question unconscious ghosts from our past that might hover between us and an accurate perception of the beauty of our partner. Working through our childhood and previous relational hurts gives us a clearer vision of our present adult relationship.

Practically, we must refocus on the positive aspects of our lover's body and soul and ignore some of the less essential parts.

We can ask our partner to remedy some of the less attractive things that are easily fixed like shaving his hairy neck or visiting a dentist more frequently or making time to exercise as a couple. Prioritizing the relationship, with time spent together doing new things, actually releases the hormone dopamine, creating exciting feelings similar to when we fall in love. Making love stimulates the release of the brain chemical oxytocin, which generates feelings of bonding. Touch connects us; orgasm cements our desire to be together. Clients often tell me that they don't feel attracted and hence don't do the things lovers do. But actually, intentional behaviors create and re-create feelings of attraction.

Does This Bed Make Me Look Fat?

For the purposes of this chapter, I have limited the discussion to women who fear rejection based on their assessment of their own diminished attraction. It weighs mightily on their minds that some men are critical, and regardless of the reason, some men do stop feeling attracted to their less than perfect wives. Life and body changes have to be met with personal integrity in order to maintain the self-confidence for ongoing sensual and sexual exchange. We have to be okay with the mirror's answer that we are no longer (or never had been) the fairest of them all.

No other aspect of attractiveness seems to interfere with women's libido as much as their feeling overweight. "I feel too fat to have sex" is an incredibly common complaint in my office. I've never really had a woman grumble that she felt too unattractive to enjoy sex once it is actually happening. She might have felt too old to attract a partner, but once she's with him, those insecurities do not seem to be as prominent or interfere as much with her desire.

Weight, unfortunately, is inescapably entwined with sexual attractiveness in our culture, and judgment is harsh toward the heavy woman. I have heard grossly obese older men criticize their wives, with no self-awareness or self-consciousness regarding their own attractiveness. (Certainly in the upcoming generation the double standard is disappearing in many ways, but only to be replaced by impossible standards of physical attractiveness for both genders.)

In his classic book *Weight, Sex, and Marriage*, Richard Stuart wrote, "The prejudice against overweight people doesn't end with the teenage [teasing] years and females continue to be the focus of discrimination. Although overweight men may be accepted on the basis of intelligence, financial status, or professional achieve-ment, overweight women are still judged primarily—even by other women—on their appearance." Similarly, Tracy Rose points out in her article "Weightism—How to Deal with Unfair Prejudice Against Obese People," that people assume that some-one who is overweight is also "lazy, cynical, unclean, ignorant, and out of control."

Overweight women do face true rejection on many levels in our culture. Objective measures about whether someone is over-weight, however, have little bearing on this sexual dilemma. Women often let a little, omnipotent machine—the dreaded scale—dispense judgment about their character. One tiny pound more than some magic number in their head can doom them to having a bad day. The number decides whether they are good or bad, worthy or not, sexy or not. That number—and not their body—tells them whether to feel desire.

Whether her partner actually despises her fat or she has become permeated by the cultural hatred of fatness, a woman internalizes those feelings. The result: a poor body image. Then, in an effort to rid herself of such toxic feelings, she projects them back onto her partner. Asking a partner the impossible-to-answer-and-stay-connected question "Do I look fat?" is only one way she does this. True or not, she sees him as hating her imperfect, "fat" body. Since a woman's desire is often responsive, she cannot feel his desire through what she imagines is his hatred of her heaviness. Her sexual desire is jeopardized by a looping mechanism of hatred over fat.

Certainly being overweight does not have to mean being unattractive or feeling unsexy. I know large women who are filled with joie de vivre, date easily and frequently, enjoy sex, and feel uninhibited about their bodies. I know men who love women of all sizes.

But for those who struggle unhappily with weight, it's a confounding problem. They may know how to eat properly, but food has become an easy anesthetic to deal with emotional highs and lows. Eating seems to keep them steady. And while there might have been specific reasons why overeating began, "once overeating is well-established," emphasizes Stuart, "it usually becomes a psychological symptom that emerges in response to any and every problem."

Food and sex both nurture our body's primitive natural needs. Primarily, overweight women are out of touch with their body's messages of hunger and satiety and often end up denying themselves the natural pleasure of food in ordinary amounts by dieting or purging. A low-libido woman blaming her fat for the reason she has no libido is similarly out of touch with her need for sexual pleasure and orgasm.

New research, as related by former Food and Drug Administration commissioner David Kessler in *The End of Overeating*, also indicates that some people are more vulnerable to our culture's increased offerings of hyperpalatable foods (sugar on fat on salt), increased food cues (restaurants on every corner, food commercials), and increased sly behavioral modification ("eat more now!") from the food industry. Drs. Eric Westman, Stephen Phinney, and Jeff Volek, authors of the *The New Atkins for the New You* argue—contrary to what we've believed and have been taught—that the "chief culprit in America's expanding waistlines is *not* fat but sugar . . ." (emphasis added). Due to the prior prevailing expert advice, women have been getting fatter eating low-fat diets when we should have been eating low-carbohydrate diets. Being overweight has many causes that can be completely unrelated to sex or marriage but can have a residual effect on self-esteem and libido.

Some women have a psychological reason for their eating habits or weight. If you're self-conscious or your judgment about your weight interferes with your sexual freedom and libido, it might be useful to explore the ways you may be using food or weight gain to assert what you're unwilling to say or are unconscious about feeling. For instance, in an earlier chapter we saw that a client's postnuptial weight gain was a defense she was using to avoid sex as a result of early memories of having been molested. The committed sexual relationship of her marriage triggered old feelings and she unconsciously gained weight to keep her safe from unwanted touch. Anxious about emotional and sexual closeness, she may unconsciously be using rolls of fat to literally keep others distant.

Food can also be a substitute for affection and love. For example, a wife—unhappy about her life and the quality of her marriage—turns to food to obtain comfort. For another woman, life's burdens feel too big and relationships have proved too untrustworthy, so her mass helps her feel like a more substantial presence in the world. Maybe weight gain is angry retaliation; she believes her previously idealized partner has become purposely malicious and hurtful so she "gets back" at him by getting fat. And sometimes overeating can be a form of self-punishment or martyrdom; an overweight woman may arrange her life to be all-giving to her family, while she herself is simultaneously deprived and overindulged at her own hand.

Heaviness can represent a test: love me no matter what and prove to me that nothing I do will make you reject me. Some women gain weight in an unconscious attempt to protect their relationship. Fat protects them from the interest of other men and relieves them of sexual dilemmas and decisions. Becoming overweight can be the remnant of childhood rebellion toward a parent's narcissistic desire for a slim child. In marriage, the spouse is now assigned a similar role—whether distorted or not—of monitoring food intake; eating in defiance of his control regardless of her real hunger or happiness is a way to separate and to feel autonomous. On the other hand, sometimes food becomes the substitute for the loving touch a partner denies her.

It's All My Fault (or Is It?)

Emily, married for twenty-three years, entered therapy complaining that she was too fat to enjoy sex. In her elastic clothes, more suited for the gym than for going out for the day, I could tell that beneath Emily's dumpy appearance was a sharp and searching mind.

Emily explained that she had gained weight right after she got married. When she and her husband were dating and early in the marriage, she'd been the higher-libido partner. Her husband, Max, had been in grad school and was distracted by his studies. By the second week after their honeymoon, he wanted sex only once a week.

"I was devastated. I felt like I wasn't attractive then—even though I was probably fifty pounds thinner and young! Plus to me, being married meant making three-course dinners. And I stopped going to the gym because that would mean more time away from precious hubby. He would be off at work or studying and other than work, I would be home waiting, cooking, and eating."

Emily was disappointed and confused. "I thought Max—and men in general—would want sex the minute they dropped their briefcase at the door, and here I was, a woman wanting it more. It made me feel unfeminine . . . like there was something wrong with me."

"You automatically thought it was your problem?" I asked.

"I'm sort of a sponge when it comes to assuming blame. Max didn't say there was something wrong with me or that he wasn't attracted to me. But he didn't reassure me either or explain the drop-off in his interest. I guess he didn't say anything. And none of my girlfriends had the problem; their husbands were clamoring for sex."

After several therapy sessions during which we talked about her marriage and her family of origin, I was beginning to get a clearer picture of the real issues. Aware only of how much she longed for Max, Emily had not realized she had chosen someone who would act out her dormant needs for space, someone who would be preoccupied with the important business of earning a living like her father had been. In actuality, her angry feelings were what made her feel unfeminine. She had never seen her mother get angry at her dad's many absences and so didn't know what to make of the turmoil inside. Absorbing the blame for the sexual problem relieved her of a confrontation. After all, if she spoke about her distress, her husband might confirm in words a more absolute rejection of her. So she assumed she wasn't attractive enough and wasn't as intellectual as his more compelling school friends. Gaining weight allowed her to play house and satisfy her dependency needs without confronting her need for autonomy, and it kept her a handicapped partner.

Emily had some male friends at work who couldn't believe her husband didn't want to have sex anymore. She admitted enjoying their flirtation and open sexual repartee. They told her that Max was "a broken guy" and that made her feel good about herself. "One of them openly told me it wasn't my problem," she said, "that my body was fine. My weight gain was so rapid I think I was protecting myself from really listening to what they were saying, perhaps from what they were offering. I started bringing bags of M&M's to work as some sort of pleasurable substitute for my own desires and defense against my coworkers' innuendos."

On some level, staying attractive might have imperiled the marriage. And so her increasing girth was meant (unconsciously) to protect the sanctity of the marital (albeit rather dead) bedroom. As she compared her marriage to what she might have had with her more passionate colleagues, she assuaged her disappointment with more chocolate.

Disparaging herself further, Emily cried with self-loathing, "I don't know what I was thinking. Where did I think those calories would go? When I asked my husband if he was still attracted to me, he said 'not as much,' and that was after gaining just ten pounds. Rather than his comment motivating me, I pulled the rip cord. I felt helpless and fat and rejected. I really haven't wanted sex since those first six months. I'll do it, but when my husband touches my thighs or my fat bottom, his fingers feel literally like painful, icy pinpricks, so I just try to get it over fast. I am never naked in front of him. And I won't do it except at night. I don't even masturbate anymore—I really couldn't care less about an orgasm. Fix that, if you can!" Similar to the anorexic who no longer wants dessert, she had mastered her sexual appetite into oblivion.

Many women express similar sentiments about their weight gain. "Women attempt to stifle their own desire for sex when their husbands can't or won't have intercourse," further declares Stuart in *Weight, Sex, and Marriage*. "Many apparently believe it 'hurts less' if they deliberately contribute to their own rejection by gaining weight. It's as if they're saying, 'You can't fire me, I quit!'"

Peignoirs or Pounds

It was time to ask Emily what might sound like an obvious question: "why are you here?" Did her husband start wanting sex after all these years or was she tired of the way things were?

She wasn't sure how to answer me. Her first response was to say she'd really like to be hypnotized in order to lose some weight. She knew, though, that her problems were more complicated than that. She'd seen her gynecologist about her years of depressingly low libido, and hoped he'd offer a pill to improve her mood and maybe help her lose weight. "But he promptly gave me your card and remarked that since I was nearly menopausal, I'd better get the weight off now."

Low-desire women often deny the complexity of their relationship and feelings. It may seem less conflictual to take the blame for the marital unhappiness because of their lack of sexual enthusiasm than to face their own dissatisfaction with the marriage. Like Emily, some overweight women funnel everything into one problem: they're fat. If they weren't fat, their spouse would be more loving. If they weren't fat, their children would respect them. If they weren't fat, they'd probably get that promotion. If they weren't fat, they'd have more energy to exercise. And if they weren't fat, they'd probably enjoy sex. The reduction of all problems to one solution makes life seem simpler but renders the multifaceted issues impossible to solve.

I asked Emily to think back to the beginning of her relationship with her husband and tell me about the sex. She thought for a minute and then shut her eyes to remember. "I think the sex was just so-so. He had a couple premature ejaculations, and the more I reassured him, the more he seemed annoyed with me and hung up about it. I was pretty sure that the problem would go away once we'd had quite a lot of sex, or at least the amount of sex I anticipated having. I didn't have any orgasms with him for several years. I knew I could because I had had them with my first boyfriend. I knew what made me come and I told Max. He listened, but didn't seem to be open to changing his technique."

The more she thought about it, the more she remembered oozing with eroticism early in her marriage. She wanted to wear sexy lingerie, but Max said it wasn't really his thing. She called him at work to talk dirty, but he would ask her politely to wait until he got home. Then he'd get home and start studying as if they'd never had a sexy conversation. She once tried giving him a blow job and he acted ticklish. "I remember feeling a strange sense of badness afterward," she added. "It was so confusing."

Maybe her higher desire was counter-stereotypical but her confusion seemed to be a mask for what was right in front of her but painful to see. Emily was simply more erotic and sexually charged than Max. Many women in my practice claim low libido only to reveal after a few sessions that their marital relations are too staid to get excited about, that they are far more sexually expert than their husbands. This too felt unfeminine to Emily because she had an old-fashioned assumption that the man should know more and want more sexually than the woman.

I asked her if she ever thought about leaving Max.

"I stay because I love him. I always have and probably always will. I think at this point he loves me. And he wants some more sex now. He's not even as critical of my body as I am. It's me who doesn't want sex at all. I just find myself so disgusting." Emily's body hatred substituted for her pent-up grief and rage at her husband's previous withholding. Her weight left her too fatigued to care.

It was time to bring Max into the sessions. A drop-off of interest in sex upon leaving the altar can happen to both men and women. As noted earlier, once commitment is secured, counter-balancing needs for independence take over, sometimes instantly. And sex—the pinnacle expression of tangible connection—can be the first thing to go. In this case, it was Max who felt that need for distance.

Early in the marriage all Emily wanted was to spend time with and be close to her husband. She was a satellite around his planet and only he had real gravity. But in talking to Max, I learned that he found her homemaking, meal making, and time demands smothering. Being the center of her world seemed too big a burden. As he scrambled to get away, her weight gain eventually offered him a reasonable excuse to reject her sexually.

Emily's attempts at closeness felt suffocating to Max and any sexual instruction Emily offered seemed to insult his masculinity and his ability to perform sexually. Sadly, in order to stay with him, she had agreed with his rejection of her open gestures and turned off her sexual eagerness. Her physical hunger was a sublimation of her sexual hunger.

Now, after years of marriage, Max had grown to be more comfortable with connection, both sexual and emotional. He wasn't aggressively sexual, but he tolerated the closeness better and relayed to Emily when he wanted sex. Indeed in some ways he wasn't the same guy who had rejected her in their young marriage. Whom was she to get mad at?

Herself, she thought. But her fury made her want to eat more. I suggested that she eat less and we deal with the terrible outpouring of feelings that would come—deprivation, rage, rebellion, self-hatred, crankiness, anger at Max, regret, guilt, fear, and pain. Because a woman's sexual appetite can grow with orgasms, I also suggested that she start to masturbate again to be in control of giving herself bodily pleasurable feelings to offset the deprivation of her diet.

At first, she didn't want to try. But she wanted to heal her marriage, and at least pleasuring herself would be easier than exposing her body to Max. Then, for a while, she cried after orgasm for the many lost years of erotic pleasure. I urged her to allow Max to touch her in ways she could tolerate—back and foot massage. I challenged her resistance to the idea that she could lose weight. "You can't control the scale—that's true—but you can control your hand-to-mouth movement. Every time you resist unhealthy cravings, you weaken their power." I worked with Emily to allow herself to feel and deal with her feelings rather than use food to numb them. For his part, Max needed to learn more sensuous ways of touching and a more reassuring way of talking. Both of them had work to do, but they were on the right road to healing.

Viva La Dark Rose

Elida was able to emigrate to the United States after winning the Cuban immigration lottery. Short, compact, and dark-skinned, in the eyes of her husband, Enrico, she was a lovely, sexual creature. Her modest weight gain kept her, not him, from feeling desire.

When she was single, nightlife in America meant drinking and dancing. But married to Enrico, a Hispanic immigrant from Mexico, Elida was bored and burdened by their seven-day workweek as they tried to get ahead. Educated in bookkeeping and project management respectively in their home countries, they had taken menial jobs while they learned English, and worked long hours just to make ends meet. They came to see me because their marriage was unsatisfying to both of them. Enrico longed for the sensual woman he married and Elida was burdened by the financial realities of their life together.

"Eli was so sexy when I met her," Enrico began. "I thought her skin was intoxicating. My dark flower."

Not so different from age-old racism in the United States, Cubans too classed people by the tone of their skin. "In Cuba," Elida told me, "my skin was too dark and so I was ugly. Rico flattered me and made me feel beautiful for the first time. But now there is no time for pretty words. All I think about is work."

Prompting Elida, I asked, "When you and Enrico used to make love, what would you think of?"

"Oh my God, I think of all kinds of things. Sometimes of nothing but his breath in my hair . . ." Elida began wistfully, but catching herself, she scolded, "Rico loves to make love. He thinks of love, love, and more love all the time. Sometimes I think I've married a boy not a man."

I teased her in order to take some of the sting out of her words about Enrico. "Elida, I know many men who only think of making love for many, many years. Even when they are old."

"Rich men, American men, men that can afford such thoughts." Elida harrumphed.

"You sound so hard, Eli. Haven't you time for love at all anymore?" asked Enrico plaintively.

"I love you, Rico. You know I do," she replied more passionately. "But anyway, I am too fat now for loving." And she added in a colder voice, "You should find some skinny American woman to waste your love on."

With evident compassion, Enrico tried to help me appreciate

his wife's feelings. "I know she loves me, Laurie, but she thinks loving with her body will take time away from our dreams. And she has it in her head I want some American girl at work. Yes, Eli has more weight now, but she is just as beautiful to me. Besides, I don't trust skinny women—they can't cook." He joked and smiled toward his wife.

Elida simply looked away and said nothing. Enrico continued: "When I try to wrap my arms around her, she pushes me away and says, 'Don't touch my stomach.' When I try to tell her she is beautiful, she accuses me of being a flirt and then is crazy jealous."

Barely deigning to change her posture, Elida accused in a tight voice, "Mrs. Laurie, he danced with this woman at the work party. I see the way he wants this skinny bitch."

"It's not true," protested Enrico. "We all dance—everyone with everyone—it is part of my culture. I don't want anyone but my wife, and she doesn't want me. I have eyes only for her, but Eli doesn't think Eli is beautiful. She is afraid I am just like her father."

Hoping to unlock some of her closed-off feelings, I asked Elida to tell me about her father and her life in Cuba. She sighed, then told an excruciating story about her father, who had left her mother when she, Elida, was small, bringing economic devastation to the family. He loved women and parties; Elida often heard him and her mother fight. Sometimes her father would come home drunk and angry. Later Elida would hear them having angry sex. She feared for her mother's safety. Her father called her mother despicable names, taunting her that he loved other women because she was ugly and dark. Fairer-skinned, he had come from a higher-class family. When he finally left, Elida was glad. But then the family had no income, and even though her mother took in laundry and sewing, they were often hungry. Elida left home at fifteen and married the first boy she found, only to find out he was "no good."

Enrico reached over to touch her while she spoke. While she cried softly, she allowed him to pull her to him but did not sink into his embrace.

Elida's inner world held parts of her parents that made sexual desire conflictual. The more we worked in treatment, the more clear it became that she feared repeating the dangerous themes of her childhood, including her mother's dependency and submissive sexuality that had allowed her father to dominate the family. Most immediately, Elida's feelings of not being attractive were a way to identify and connect with her mother, whom she missed. Even though her husband had awakened the sleeping beauty within her early in their relationship, she was afraid that his appetite for beauty would always keep him looking for someone more attractive. And his power to call her beautiful left her at his mercy. Enrico's love of a good time and sex reminded her of her father, both attracting and frightening her. Fearful, she held her eroticism down. Punishing them both for loving feelings that might get out of control, she pushed them both to work harder. Her father did not like chubby women, so in some ways her weight protected her from old feelings about his seductive potency. She insulated the party girl inside with a bit of padding because of the ways her sexual feelings kept her connected to her treacherous, promiscuous father.

In therapy, Elida learned how to separate Enrico's warmth and erotic love for her from the sadomasochistic model of her parents' connection. Seeing that her lack of libido was unconsciously meant to punish her mother for having sexual desire for a dangerous man, she started to allow herself to relax into Enrico's tenderness. She also began to see that her sexual disconnect from Enrico increased his vulnerability to and likelihood of affairs rather than encouraging his desire for her. Talking about her fear of replicating her childhood replaced the "fat" talk that had hidden her central issues around intimacy.

Our bodily self-image is tied up with the way our families viewed our attractiveness and our development. I was a tomboy, but my German grandfather thought I was enchanting. He taught me to say in German the words to a popular song of his day: "I love you, and to me, you are beautiful." He would say it to me over and over. Though I was awkward and chubby, I felt like the most beautiful girl in the world. As we've discussed, if a father delights in a mother and expresses joy in his daughter's beauty, she can more easily transcend the cultural demand for bodily perfection. When Mama warmly accepted Daddy's arms around a slightly chubby middle—with no comments about dieting—the girl learns that love and affection are not tied to thinness. If you had parents who accepted the various losses of aging with equanimity and humor, then you are not afraid that your essential beauty will be compromised as your youth fades. Without that positive heritage, we must work harder to escape our culture's pressure that only the physically perfect are sexy or sexual.

Help Yourself

1. What messages surrounding your attractiveness did you learn from childhood?

2. Describe your most attractive features.

3. How does weight impact your sexual desire?

4. If you are overweight, does your weight have meaning beyond your enjoyment of food?

5. Are there parts of your body that are off-limits when you make love?

6. Imagine a body acceptable enough for you to enjoy all sex offers. What would happen if you allowed your current body to be fully acceptable?

CHAPTER THIRTEEN

The Inevitable Big M

When does a woman reach her sexual peak? Trick question. If you answered thirty-five, you'd be talking about the age when a woman finally feels comfortable enough to ask for, even demand, the pleasure she wants. Our enjoyment of sex comes from a combination of physiology, emotional connection, and erotic entitlement. But a woman's hormonal peak occurs at about age eighteen to twenty, just as it does for males.[1]

Menopause, marked by one full year after our periods stop, happens when our ovaries significantly reduce hormonal production. That occurs, on average, at around age fifty-one. Our fertility ends but our sexual enjoyment doesn't have to. This natural process of aging does bring physiological changes and we may have to learn to make love in new and adaptive ways. Being open to change is insurance against a sexual shutdown. Nearly all women retain the ability to have orgasms from the cradle to the grave, though with advancing age, it may take longer, require new technique, and/or multiple stimuli.

Liberated from the fear of pregnancy, women may find menopause to be a time of personal freedom, and that can contribute to our sexual pleasure. We can stop caring so much about what people think of us. We can stop focusing so much on our stomachs and relax into sensuality during sex. And we can stop propping up our husbands, lovers, children, parents, and what can feel like the whole damn world. We can say yes to ourselves. We can say what we think and get rid of pent-up, held-back emotions. We don't have to put up with poor treatment from anyone. We can tell our lovers to go down and get busy. We can come into our own. While waning hormones mean a physiological change, our minds can make this a very sexy time.

Flashing Hot

Many of us experience a variety of symptoms like tiredness, hot flashes, night sweats, insomnia, forgetfulness, irritability, vaginal dryness, and lowered libido. About 20 percent of women are mercifully without symptoms, so don't compare yourself to your best girlfriend who seems to be going through the change easily.[2] Additionally, indicators may appear years before actual menopause. Thirty-one percent of us experience lower libido and a change in sexual responsiveness during the two or three years leading up to the end of our periods.[3]

Let's take a closer look at two hormones that impact our sexual experience—estrogen and testosterone—and what happens to them during menopause.

Lower estrogen can cause a loss of vaginal health. Our vaginas become drier, and can even become smaller.[4] Our genital tissue can look pale, and become thin and more subject to tearing. Thinning tissue makes us more prone to urinary tract infections (UTIs) and painful sex. Unfortunately, pain leads women to avoid sex. Since orgasms and the rigor of sexual foreplay and intercourse could bring healing blood flow to the genital tissue, a vicious cycle ensues.

Testosterone governs the physiological feelings of desire in both genders. Dona Caine-Frances, R.N., sex therapist, and author of *Managing Menopause Beautifully*, says a woman's levels are down by half by menopause, falling steadily with age. Sexual desire as a physiologic push grows nonexistent. As women, we have never had the levels of this desire-making sex dope that men experience. For instance, the normal range of healthy male testosterone levels is between 270 and 1,070 nanograms per deciliter of blood,[5] whereas women range merely from 5 to 70 ng/dl.[6] A man at the lower ranges, perhaps 200 to 300 nanograms, will often experience low desire. He thinks about sex only once a week, doesn't want it after a fight with his wife, and experiences trouble with his erections. For a woman, the serum blood level and her free testosterone level (the amount bioavailable for desire) do not completely correlate as directly as men's do to feelings of desire, but the difference is worth bearing in mind. Women with high levels can still have low libido and vice versa. A postmenopausal woman with lower testosterone levels can find herself in a brand-new relationship and roar with libido. Adequate testosterone also promotes a sense of well-being and depression is often caused by its depletion. We also know from studies that testosterone replacement along with estrogen in women who have surgical menopause (removal of ovaries) does improve libido.[7]

Dependable lovemaking routines can suddenly change too. What worked before may not work now. Let's say a couple's lovemaking typically started with him getting her aroused, her arousal getting him hard, and his erection getting her even more excited. That pattern of excitement is thrown off if step one—her initial arousal—takes much longer than it used to. Men who might have defined a woman's wet vagina as the definitive sign that she's hot to trot may feel disappointed at that lack of an obvious signal. They misread their lover's body as saying no, in much the same way that women can misread erectile dysfunction to mean their husband isn't attracted to them anymore. Artificial lubricant could easily be worked into a familiar routine, and shouldn't signal a shortcoming on either partner's part. The menopausal woman confronted with aging anatomy needs a sturdy sense of her value in spite of technical difficulties.

The aging process can feel devastating to a woman who defines herself as a head turner. If desire has meant the ability to elicit interest from men—i.e., being desirable—then being ignored or passed over can hit a woman's ego hard. And we've been told for aeons that being sexy means how we look rather than what we think and feel in our hearts. Hopefully, by menopause, we have learned how to respect ourselves as owner and manufacturer of desire, not as simply an enticement for others.

Hot flashes or night sweats and increased anxiety can ruin sleep and leave a woman tired. Virginia told me she felt like "a shadow of her former self." Madison reported that even with two cold showers a day, she sweated so much that her husband asked if she was allergic to him. For most women, these are the most disruptive symptoms and the reason they seek medical relief.

Depression and distractibility are common. Forgetfulness can worry an aging woman, making her fear that she's losing her mental prowess at the same time as her physical vitality. All of these symptoms can make sex less desirable. Psychologically, a woman who has had good libido all her life may miss her body's easy push of desire and response to stimulation. At sixty, Susan expressed her dismay by saying, "Why bother? If it's this difficult, I'm just not sure I want to go to the trouble."

Is Hormone Therapy Dangerous?

In the 1960s, hormone therapy (HT) seemed to be the fountain of youth. With hope of proving its protective benefits against heart disease and osteoporosis, a randomized, controlled, fifteen-year study called the Women's Health Initiative (WHI) was started to assess its risks and benefits. Because of the surprising and unexpected results, the study was prematurely ended in 2002. Preliminary results seemed to indicate that taking hormones was dangerous, increasing the risks of breast cancer, heart disease, and stroke.

Throughout the country, many women were taken immediately off their HT by their doctors. Health practitioners became anxious about potential legal liability if they kept women on or put new patients on HT. In the summer of 2002, my counseling center, Awakenings, was inundated by calls from menopausal women previously on HT, anxiously questioning why they suddenly had no sexual desire. Lower desire is a natural side effect of not having enough hormones.

The North American Menopausal Society (NAMS) and the American College of Gynecologists and Obstetricians have reviewed the limitations of the WHI study in retrospect. First, women subjects had been older than typical menopausal women by about ten years and had significantly more health risks when started on the hormones. Further analysis, though, showed that younger women closer to menopause experienced only minimal risk of increased coronary heart disease. The time when women could or should receive medical intervention affects the relative risks of treatment. Officially, both organizations decided that, for most women, when using HT close to the time of menopause, the benefits related to long-term health and short-term symptom relief outweigh the risks. Using it for as short a time as necessary (long-term use is defined as greater than five years) also reduces risk.[8]

Also, in the WHI study, only one type of estrogen, alone or combined with one type of progesterone, was studied. The oral replacement of estrogen and progesterone used in the study, rather than the alternative transdermal (through the skin) delivery, meant that potentially two to three times more hormone was needed in order for the right amount to get into the blood stream.[9] Pills also had to be metabolized through the liver, increasing the risk of blood clots and stroke.[10] Now, in response to our better understanding of the risks, lower doses or micronized doses of HT as well as better delivery systems with patches and creams and gels have been developed.[11]

All women need an evaluation from their physician to determine their particular risks. Those with breast or endometrial cancer, cardiovascular disease, thromboembolic disorders, and active liver disease may not be candidates for HT.

Should you supplement with hormones? Will they improve your sexual desire? Are they safe for your particular health history? Why would you decide for or against HT? Like Louise below, these are questions that every woman struggles with.

Time to Spare but Out of Sync

At fifty-one, Louise had had a good marriage, but her older husband's early retirement was creating a bit of havoc. "I feel nothing," she said of her sex life, dressed in coordinating active wear and sporting a cropped haircut. "And I feel like I've reached an age that I don't have to fuss with looking or acting sexy. I'm comfortable with who I am. I know my husband feels cheated that I'm not so interested in filling our golden years with lovemaking and wandering naked through our beach house. But criminy, I don't want to do that. I've got things I want to do."

Louise's husband, Henry, had retired after a busy career and now had time to spare to be relational and, as she put it, to be underfoot. He'd wake up and excitedly ask her what they were going to do that day. "Nothing!" she'd want to say. She already had her day's agenda and it didn't include entertaining a husband. Particularly as night sweats dominated her night's agenda and left her tired and irritable.

Sexually, his desire hadn't diminished, though she mentioned that the time it took for him to get an erection had slowed down. "He still really wants it," she claimed. "But not me. I take forever to come. And most of the time I just don't care. Sure, I want the marriage to be good and all that. But I just don't want sex. It hasn't always been like this either. I used to want it. But now, not so much. I've told him I'll just give him a blow job whenever he wants it, but I could do without intercourse. I don't want to go to bed with all the stuff dripping out of me. It's hard enough to go to sleep. I wouldn't tell him that, though. And frankly, it takes him forever to get hard, which is a real drag."

How was intercourse feeling? "Not good would be an understatement. I'm always tight and it often hurts."

Had Henry taken her up on her offer of oral sex whenever he wanted? "Obviously not or I wouldn't be here. Whaddaya got, Laurie? Can you get me some of those little blue pills?"

I can't prescribe medication, but I explained that while Viagra helps men with blood-flow difficulties to produce erections, it doesn't do a thing about "wanting." Pharmaceutical companies are frantically working on a female desire pill and will probably make a large fortune if successful, but so far, there is no herbal supplement or manufactured drug that has been shown to reliably increase desire other than hormonal supplementation.

I believed Louise about her body's sensations. She still had her ovaries but had a hysterectomy earlier in life because of fibroids. She was a candidate for estrogen-only supplementation using a patch or gel. Progesterone is necessary only for women who have an intact uterus to protect the organ from cancer. Her gynecologist did a thorough examination, including assessing her family history of breast cancer and cardiac disease. Generally healthy, Louise did not have any particular cardiovascular risk factors like obesity, high blood pressure, diabetes, smoking, or history of blood clots. She and the doctor had already discussed nonhormonal ways to manage hot flashes, like limiting caffeine, a healthful diet, supplementing with omega-3 fatty acids, avoiding spicy foods, alcohol, and tobacco, and maintaining a regular exercise regimen.

Her gynecologist prescribed an estradiol patch, a bioidentical estrogen, to be changed midweek to help relieve her hot flashes. Bioidentical hormones are chemical copies of those found in your body. Estradiol, micronized progesterone, and testosterone are all bioidentical hormones. The WHI was done using conjugated equine estrogen or estrogen made from pregnant horses with a slightly different microbiology than the body's molecules. Claims are being made that bioidentical hormones are without risk or more natural. All hormones are synthetic—compounded chemically and produced in mass quantity.[12] Some bioidentical hormones are FDA-approved and covered by insurance, but others are compounded as creams by special pharmacies whose integrity should be verified by your physician. These are frequently not covered by insurance. In a European study of eighty thousand women, some evidence did suggest that micronized progesterone is safer for breast tissue than the progesterone studied in the WHI and other nonbioidentical hormones. Also, transdermal estradiol appears to have less blood-clotting risk than oral estrogen of any kind. But none of these studies were randomized and controlled, so more research is necessary.[13]

Hormones often take two to four weeks to achieve full effect. If a woman does not experience complete resolution of her symptoms, estradiol comes in a variety of doses that can be adjusted to help her. Louise also required additional prescription vaginal estrogen tablets to ease her discomfort. By thickening the canal walls and increasing blood flow, estrogen makes the vagina more elastic and less susceptible to tearing. Vaginal estrogen can also come as a vaginal cream or ring, but Louise didn't like the mess of a cream. With regular stretching both by herself in the shower using her own fingers and through intercourse, she was able to keep her vagina supple enough to avoid pain.

I further suggested an artificial lubricant. Typically, I recommend an unscented silicone-based lubricant. This provides the best glide without becoming gummy and without being absorbed. Olive oil can be used in a pinch. It has the added benefit of a decent taste during oral sex.

I also knew that if we could eliminate some of the emotional barriers and relationship complexities that were involved in Louise's low-libido mix, we would at least get a clearer picture of what aspects were purely physiological. All life transitions—getting married, having a baby, retiring—need a renegotiation to balance closeness and distance between two people.

Louise told me about two problems regarding their new arrangement. The first was too much togetherness. She felt crowded both outside and inside the bedroom. For women at any age, being penetrated can feel like the ultimate invasion or takeover. Some welcome the sensation, while others who need more psychological space find intercourse more challenging. I wondered if she was using her words, power, and negotiation skills to find the right balance of time and literal space with her husband in this relatively happy relationship. To be satisfying to her, physical joining couldn't feel like it was crowding her, interfering with her agenda, or ignoring her needs.

Like Mother, Like Daughter?

Louise's second problem was that she had stopped seeing herself as a sexual being. When does a woman become a crone? Often when she starts to identify with how she saw her mother. We may never accurately perceive our mothers, and perhaps their sexuality even less so. An overtly sexual mother threatens the child's fantasy perspective of being the center of Mommy's world.[14] Adult desire pulls Mother away to the exciting father or other, and our childhood self-centeredness suffers. It is proof positive that she exists not only for us but also for herself. So we block out this aspect of our mothers. At some point, though, we age into our mother's shoes.

"When I look in the mirror," Louise admitted, "I no longer see just my mother's face, but I see her body. I see her sagging breasts and her flattening bottom. Being sexy and adventurous belonged to my other body."

By her own admission, she was beginning to act like a prude. "I reject Henry's public innuendos because sex feels more and more private to me. He wants me to still tease him and, I suppose, to wear sexy clothes, but it just doesn't seem to fit our station in life to act—or dress—like teenagers," said Louise.

Her mind agreed with her body. Sexy belonged to that different body.

Louise's mother and father had slept in twin beds in an old white farmhouse. As she grew up, life had been filled with hard work, and Louise remembered her mother as a no-nonsense laundress and cook. Throughout her childhood, Louise never heard a word from her mother about sex, and she imagined her now-widowed mother as asexual. Perhaps her mother had never been interested in sex, but perhaps she'd had a healthy libido and simply chosen never to speak to Louise about anything related to sex. The problem for Louise was her sliding toward an identity that ostensibly excluded the pleasures of the flesh.

She didn't want sex, but she did want physical connection. "I still want to be touched. I like to be petted really—my head stroked, my feet rubbed, my shoulders kneaded. But Henry hasn't ever wanted to do that. Or he gets aroused and then we have to have sex. So I just forget all of it."

Challenging her, I asked why she didn't stand up for her need as fervently as her husband was arguing for a continued sex life.

"Being demanding seems the opposite of being feminine to me. Yet I resent that he won't fulfill the physical needs I have, and so I suppose I withhold giving him what he wants. I don't want Henry to be turned off by my assertiveness, but I don't want to turn him on either . . . what a conundrum!"

Louise had seen her mother as having a quiet, practical strength, but her mother had been the first one to jump up at the table to fetch Louise's father more water. Louise had been a pleaser in her marriage too, always the first to back down from her side of the argument. She and her husband's roles had been clearly defined until recently. In order to have a more intimate relationship and be true to herself, Louise was going to have to risk stating what she needed: more physical affection, daytimes to herself, and maybe even to say, "Make your own damn sandwich." We talked about femininity being about respecting intuition, valuing *the way* things happened as much as *that* they happened, and compassionate strength that cherished others and the self. She needed to redefine what it meant to be a woman by adding firmness about her own needs.

Sexually, she needed to have a strong voice about her preferences in order for the rare moments of her desire to result in the very best possible experience—now more than ever. Because her body was changing, things she and Henry had done in their early years felt uncomfortable. Because she held to her mother's mold that equated femininity with compliance, she hadn't spoken up about the need for change.

Everything Changes

Later, I asked Louise what her husband's slower erections meant to her. "Henry always had good strong erections before and we could have easy, playful sex. If he wanted a quickie, I'd be up for it. Now there is no such thing as a quickie. Sex means a big production." We talked about flexible lovemaking patterns, where Henry might sometimes take responsibility for his own stimulation, as she did for herself in years gone by, and come to Louise ready again for a genuine quickie.

A man's instant erection can also signify to a woman her own desirability. What power her attractiveness had to levitate his penis from afar! She was an enchantress. Now that his physiological changes were coinciding with her sense of being less desirable, she felt she had lost her magic. She and Henry were reduced to having mundane sex—or no sex at all. Chivers's research on pornography showed that women were physiologically aroused by all kinds of nudity and sexual scenes—including those of bonobo monkeys mating—all except for a naked, flaccid man walking on a beach.[15]

A Male Problem Too?

Often by middle age, men need just about as much physical stimulation to get aroused as women have needed all along. Without the tangible cue of an erection, however, women can be less aroused even if they were never particularly conscious of having felt excited by the sight of an erect phallus. Unfortunately, a woman's misinterpretation can make both parties feel misunderstood. He feels less sure of his potency to arouse her and she feels less attractive. Accepting our partners' aging and changing body allows other cues to signal desire.

In his book *Rekindling Desire*, Barry McCarthy says sex stops when a couple ages most frequently because the man withdraws, and 90 percent of the time he stops pursuing because of his own anxiety over his erections. Waning potency or low testosterone can mean partner problems that derail sexuality. For the record, men with low normal or below normal levels of testosterone also experience low desire. If a man has low testosterone, he acts like a lot of the women we've discussed when it comes to how life's stresses impact his desire. Get in a fight with him and he won't want sex that night. Worried over Johnny's troubles at school, he won't want sex for a week. I often see couples with a low-testosterone husband. Because it is so countercultural, their wives have suffered years of damage to their self-esteem keeping this painful reality secret. "How can I say my husband never wants me? I'm so ashamed to be the only one at a cocktail party whose husband isn't pawing her. I feel like an ugly freak," relates the very-not-ugly Emily. I always tell these men, "Do not pass go. Do not see a therapist first. Go directly to your physician and have your hormones tested."

Testosterone doesn't cause cancer, but because prostate cancers are fed by this hormone, men need to have a digital rectal exam and blood work to monitor their current prostate-specific antigen (PSA) levels (cancer increases this antigen in the blood) before starting supplementation. No exceptions!

Men are fortunate in that, if the root of their problem is hormonal, replacement nearly always restores desire. Middle age brings diseases and medications that affect desire and erections and often men face problems for the first time at this juncture. Fortunately, Viagra (or Levitra or Cialis) nearly always works to restore erections. But should supplementation fail or a disease like prostate cancer strike, men too must find eroticism that is deeper than the body.

If testosterone is not the issue but psychological factors are causing a man to slow down or shut down his sexuality, the trouble can be much deeper psychologically. Low testosterone can be one cause of depression, but treatment with SSRIs will slacken desire and slow orgasm. Emotional ambivalence about closeness can cause low libido. Perhaps these men fear being swallowed up or controlled. Giving themselves over to their wives feels dangerous to some men; penetration can symbolically seem more like putting their private parts into a giant trap. Just like women, they can fear that their feelings of lust and need subject them to possible rejection and abandonment, so their solution becomes feel less, need less.

Finding a New Balance

While homemaking is a difficult and arduous task, it's rare that a family expresses gratitude commensurate with the work. As a whole, our culture doesn't value the contribution of caring for others in the same way that we admire achievement in the workplace, and a woman must struggle to know her significance in the lives of her family. In earlier times, Louise felt dependent on the relationship to bring her happiness—the highlight of her day was her husband coming home from work. With two grown children doing well in their lives, she was satisfied with the results of her life's purpose of homemaking during their earlier family years. Now she had found a new direction to express her creativity through art, and with the right communication, Henry began to respect her limits. As a result, she found sharing her body easier.

When Louise ended therapy she summarized what had changed. "I'm more my own person now. I can do what I want. My time's my own and I'm involved with the community and with my art in deeper ways than were possible before. I think that my separateness from Henry has kept him on his toes. Now he's often at home waiting for me to arrive. We've flip-flopped and I like the fact that his world focuses more on me. It makes me feel wanted and important. Some of our earlier problems have gone away. I don't feel like he takes me for granted anymore. Maybe both of us realize that life isn't forever. And sex has become sweeter if less frequent.

"I don't think I expect sex to solve problems that it wasn't meant to solve. When I was younger, I loaded it with expectations about his love and appreciation for me. Even if sex was pleasurable at the time, if he didn't act romantic, I would feel unsatisfied. Now I can have easier sex without trying to read meaning into every encounter. I accept that he loves me in many ways. He has provided for me. He notices when the carpet needs tacking down. He does little things around the house that I would never get to. I can now count all of it as love." At last, sex was unburdened from being the sole bearer of her husband's feelings.

"I've understood that his erection or lack of one," Louise added, "is not a reflection of how he feels about me. I'm willing to give him more time and stimulation during sex. And I've told him foot rubs are mandatory while we watch TV together in the evening."

Older and Bolder

Unlike Louise, Magna didn't struggle with being too compliant, at least not any longer. In head, out mouth was her new policy. "Screw it. I'll say what I want at this age. If people don't like me, guess what? I don't care. I dumped my husband several years back. He'd been a jerk for so long and I thought, 'You know, I've had quite enough of you, you're outta here!' My adult children nearly stood up and cheered. They'd had enough of him too. I only wish I hadn't subjected them to a man like him when they were little. Now I've found a great guy and would love to have some wild sex with him. But there is no big bang left in this old broad. My clit is dead, I think."

At sixty-four, Magna might have teased about being old, but she was younger at heart than many women I talk with. Dumping her abusive husband renewed her energy for life and love and she had found a kind and satisfying partner. Christiane Northrup, acclaimed author and physician, writes that two things block experiencing life's pleasure: anger and self-doubt.[16] Magna had spent the better part of life seething with resentment and not knowing how to change. Menopause clarified her direction. Along with the root cause of her anger, she ditched her libido-draining patterns—giving too much to others was replaced by a more appropriate sense of entitlement. Fighting for all that life had to offer, she wanted sexual satisfaction. But she was having some technical problems.

"I've tried it all, Laurie. I bought the 'rabbit' [a vibrator with a special clitoral stimulator], and James has worn my poor nub out trying to get some reaction out of me. I've lotioned and potioned up and all I get is a little ping—sort of a mild rise rather than a reverberating climax like I used to have. I'm so desperate, I'll do whatever you say to do. I'd like to try testosterone, but my doctor sent me to you first. I don't care if I go bald and sprout a beard if it will bring back some feeling."

Testosterone is not FDA-approved for women, and authoritative studies have verified neither its safety for anything longer than six months used in conjunction with estrogen, nor its effect on the heart, breasts, and uterus. But it is often tried off-label to help with sexual desire problems. Magna's physician prescribed a specially compounded testosterone cream from one of our local reputable compounding pharmacies. Testim and Androgel are FDA-approved medications for men that are sometimes used at significantly lower doses when prescribed for women. Again, the liver is spared harm because the chemical is absorbed straight into the bloodstream through the skin. Common side effects of testosterone are hair growth on the body and acne. Less common side effects include voice deepening, weight gain, and possible hair thinning on the head. Hair growth can be tweezed away. Lots of women past forty are plucking a stray hair or two, but electrolysis might become necessary. Levels are checked at specific intervals for safety and compared to a woman's individual feelings of desire.

Some data show that using a testosterone patch on surgically induced menopausal women resulted in two additional love-making sessions a month.[17] Obviously, if a couple wishes for an increase of sex to four times a week, this is a poor result. But if it means a couple goes from making love once a month to almost every week, it can produce much more happiness. However, using oral testosterone can lower one's good HDL cholesterol. Injectable and implanted tablets of testosterone may raise the hormone level too high. All androgen supplementation carries some risk and should be evaluated carefully with your physician.

After three months on testosterone, Magna returned and told me that she had had two good orgasms, but each had taken up to an hour to achieve, with lots of stimulation. The intermittent nature of her orgasms still had her worried. But it was good news to me and I believed that if she had two, she could have more. Many premenopausal women need at least forty-five minutes of general stroking and clitoral stimulation for satisfaction. As I've said, good postmenopausal sex can take significantly longer for both genders, and relaxing about that fact would lessen the counterforce of anxiety that stifles orgasm.

While Magna said she had tried everything, I wanted to make sure that she had systematically tried techniques I knew helped create the best opportunity for a more powerful orgasm. I call the following technique "sexual baseball." First, she needed to start with an erotic mind-set and enough clitoral stimulation. Through touching or vibration, build toward orgasm but stop short on the first two tries or "strikes."

In between strikes, she was to let her body relax for a minute or so. Then resume building sexual tension with more touching. Changing the type of touch from deep pressure to light clitoral glans friction (with lots of lubrication) would keep her mind from getting bored.

I asked her to have her boyfriend put his fingers in her vagina and tell her to alternately squeeze and relax with enough pressure that he registered the constriction. The increased muscular tension in her pelvis would change the sensation as he continued to touch her clitoris. When she relaxed her Kegel muscles (the same contraction women use to stop the flow of urine), he was to stimulate her G-spot. Yes, there is a G-spot! The G-spot is on the roof of the vagina toward her belly button when a women is lying on her back, inside the canal and below the urethra. When a partner stimulates it using a "come-hither" motion, crooking his finger and gently stroking the roof of the vagina about two to three inches inside, a woman who is not quite aroused enough may feel a sensation similar to the feeling of needing to urinate. If she feels this, he has found her G-spot, and with more arousal she will usually feel intense pleasure.

Coming closer to orgasm, she should relax and he should use very light pressure to keep her slightly on the cliff. On the third strike, he should continue stimulation to let her climax. Home run!

Previously they had rushed toward orgasm as soon as Magna felt good sensations. Psychologically, this new game changed her mind-set from how fast she could come to trying to keep from going over the edge before she was allowed. It also extended love play and increased her focus on pleasure. Her body could gather the maximum swelling, lubrication, and circulation that would maximize her orgasm. Women (and men) who struggle with any anxiety over orgasm can benefit from this game, as it turns the goal upside down. "Don't come" rather than coming becomes the aim for a short period of time.

Magna also said she liked anal touching but not penetration. For some women, the idea of anal play is anathema, but for a small percentage, anal penetration is highly enjoyable. When women have trouble reaching orgasm, they should use as many types of simultaneous stimulation as possible. Anything touching the anus should not be put in the vagina afterward in order to avoid bacterial contamination. Other erogenous zones include the neck, earlobes, fingers, toes, the small of the back, and the back of the knees. Magna's favorite way to reach orgasm became being on top for intercourse, using a small clitoral vibrator along with her boyfriend touching her anus.

Though she had tried some topical products on her own, I recommended others to see if they might boost arousal. Zestra, for example, is a herbal compound that studies have shown to increase arousal for some women. It produces a warming sensation topically similar to the tingling of sexual stimulation. My own caveat is that warming lubricants may feel like burning when used on dry, postmenopausal, vulvar tissue. Magna also tried a prescription cream containing alprostadil, which increases blood flow and can heighten orgasmic intensity. Over-the-counter nipple creams with cooling sensations increased her sensitivity and added a layer of arousal. I also recommended she talk to her physician about trying Viagra, which, as a recent study has shown, is not just for men but can help increase the power of orgasm in women who are struggling with arousal.

For some women, these commercial and pharmaceutical aids feel too artificial, but Magna had already accepted that her body's original capacity had changed. She wanted to want again. I agreed with her that most of her sexual dissatisfaction was due to hormonal depletion rather than purely psychological issues. And it took time to find a solution to all of the different issues she struggled with. Orgasms did not get easy but they resumed their intensity.

Bridgett, on the other hand, did not want any hormonal intervention. Insulin-resistant and with a family history of cardiovascular disease, she had too many risk factors for HT. Her primary complaint was that she had less libido than before menopause. Hot flashes she could live with, but sex had been an important part of her relationship and she wanted to see what could be done to boost her sexual hunger.

When a woman is motivated to increase her libido, she often accepts the assignments of sex therapy easily. I suggested that she choose an intimate time and declare it sacred against other tasks, hobbies, or occupations. After busy working lives, Bridgett and her life partner Jill's early retirement focused on physical health and de-stressing. Their special time was often early in the day, following exercise and the morning meal in their sunny breakfast room. Seeking connection to each other via mind, body, and spirit, they took turns reading passages from poetry and inspirational books. After taking a couples' class on massage, they often practiced their new skills on each other.

I encouraged Bridgett to ask for genital massage and let herself receive the gift with no expectation to return the favor at least some of the time. Jill gladly participated. While she felt selfish at first, Bridgett started to experience a new receptivity and craving for all kinds of touch. Having her hair brushed reminded her of her mother's ministrations. Slow, flat palms circling on her back were also like soothing touches from childhood. No current negotiations were allowed during their connection time. She learned to deeply rest in Jill's arms as they shared their memories of their parents, their families, their lives and accomplishments. Without the constant strain of work, they were left with more time to lavish affection on each other. Her feelings of attachment to Jill expanded as she allowed touch to emerge as an even deeper conduit of connection. They allowed each other a regression to a time when the first language of their relationship was holding, touching, and stroking. Receiving pleasure without pressure lessened her resistance to the times that their experiment turned sexual. Desire became part of the physicality that their relationship nurtured.

After several months, Bridgett told me that there was a fullness to their relationship that had not been there even when she had felt more spontaneously sexual. "I feel cared for," she explained, "on such a primitive level. Jill's willingness to give so much has filled up the places inside me where I felt ashamed of needing, where I believed I had overwhelmed my mother with my need. I've come to see my need as healthy. My sexual desire for Jill comes from a place in my heart."

Therapy can help menopausal women work through a poor body image, relational difficulties, and a constricted repertoire of sexual techniques. Your physician should be your final authority when making decisions for or against using HT. Like every stage of sexual development, menopause needs some conscious thinking and purposeful changes to make it the most fulfilling and intimate time possible.

Help Yourself

1. Discuss expectations with your partner for retirement activities and time spent together.

2. What was your mother like during menopause?

3. If you are menopausal, how has your body changed and what symptoms, if any, are you experiencing?

4. Discuss freedoms and restrictions that you feel in your sexuality at this life phase.

CHAPTER FOURTEEN

When Sex Hurts

Pain stops sexual desire cold. There's nothing like a stinging or burning sensation in the vagina to make libido evaporate. Unfortunately, women with dyspareunia—pain during intercourse—often ignore it or complain about it only to be told they should try to "relax." The problem with any kind of sexual pain is that it often gets worse if we don't discover why it's happening and what to do about it.

Maybe a woman is having trouble getting aroused, and frustrated, she tells her husband to just go ahead. Intercourse hurts and afterward she feels some burning when she goes to the bathroom. Maybe this happens a second time. A third time. Something isn't right and she knows it. A critical voice in her head tells her that she ought to enjoy sex and worries that her husband is going to notice pretty soon. She hides the pain, soldiers on, and often begins to feel guilty about her lack of enjoyment. Because of her dread of the pain, her body will not get aroused, will not lubricate or swell, and yet she rushes to have intercourse too early when any woman would find it uncomfortable. Sensibly, her body won't respond naturally because the end result hurts. Unbelievably, women with these problems continue to have sex and then describe it later as burning, sandpapery, or even like a "hot knife." By the time she gets to a doctor, this has been going on for too long. When she makes an appointment with me, she has suffered extensively, her husband has mostly given up hope, and their sex life has been derailed.

I see women with sexual pain issues referred by a doctor who hopes I can help. At first it's not always easy to figure out what's causing the problem—in mind, body, or relationship. Often the problem is physical, leaving the woman relieved it doesn't mean that she doesn't like sex or might not love her husband or any number of things that she's made up to try to make sense of it all. Together we figure out what referrals will be most helpful. If sex has stopped, the couple needs help finding ways to reconnect sensually. I help with specific sexual work-arounds so that she can have pleasure again. Occasionally I have to suggest a whole new way to have sex. Making love doesn't mean "insert penis into vagina." But couples often need permission to return to pleasurable touching when intercourse hurts. Sexual pain problems that have their roots in anxiety, however, need sex therapy combined with traditional psychotherapy to be successfully treated.

Many Kinds of Ouch

Genital pain can happen during intercourse, during stimulation and arousal, or sometimes simply during daily activities. All of it will derail sex. And all sorts of things can cause pain or irritation, many of which are easy to remedy. The following are some of the most common causes of pain and recommended treatments:

- Hygienic practices should be as gentle as possible. Really, warm water is all that is needed to clean the vulva and make a woman fresh. Sensitive women should avoid all chemical-containing feminine products like douches or scented tampons, which are unnecessary in the first place.

- What you eat can impact the health and the condition of your vulva. Foods high in oxalic acid like spinach or tomatoes produce waste crystals in urine that can irritate delicate tissues. Not that any of us should stop eating these healthy foods, but some may need to neutralize the acid with calcium citrate under a doctor's supervision. Sometimes showering off after urination can bring relief too. I highly recommend installing a shower wand in the master bathroom. While dietary changes are controversial in the medical community, many women in my practice have reported success with a low-oxalate diet.

- Women suffering from vaginal dryness should increase their consumption of omega-3 fatty acids and vitamin E to their doctor's specifications.

- Extended use of birth control pills sometimes causes vaginal dryness. Lubricants may be necessary even for young users. Vaginal estrogen may also help. A reexamination of birth control might be necessary.

- Postmenopausal women may need estrogen to make the vagina supple enough for comfortable intercourse. Even women who cannot take oral estrogen may be candidates for vaginal estrogen, as it has much less effect on their total hormonal blood levels.

- Infections from yeast or bacteria are easily cured when brought to a physician's attention. Yeast infections can linger, and while most women know to look for the white cottage-cheese-like discharge, they can also cause genital redness, itching, or pain and must be diagnosed using a pathology slide under a microscope. Dietary changes to control high blood sugar in diabetics or prediabetics may be necessary to control yeast.

- Lichen sclerosis may be caused by autoimmune disorders and looks like whitish, cigarette-paper-like, thin, easily torn skin and can be managed by steroid ointment (clobetasol).[1]

- Chronic itching can be the result of a scratch-itch cycle.[2] With proper medication, the woman can stop the unconscious nocturnal scratching that exacerbates the problem.

- An untreated sexually transmitted disease may cause all sorts of problems but can often be mitigated through treatment. For instance, herpes can be repressed through drug therapy. Gonorrhea (bacteria), chlamydia (bacteria), and trichomoniasis (parasite) can all cause pain and are treatable with antibiotics.[3]

- Reentry into a sexual relationship after childbirth can be painful. Obviously, any tearing or an episiotomy from a vaginal delivery can cause pain. Even women who've had a cesarean delivery can experience discomfort because of hormonal changes. Both cases might be eased with vaginal estrogen cream. See your gynecologist.

While I've listed only a few potential etiologies of genital pain, the causes are extensive, complicated, and, most importantly, treatable!

Ashley, nineteen, was a college sophomore who told me she was "broken." Sex hurt and she never got wet. I asked her to describe sex with her boyfriend. "Well, he gets home from classes and we lie down and do it." No foreplay, no arousal time, no orgasm for her—it took them all of five minutes. The condoms they used added further friction that irritated her vagina. Ashley had been labeled dysfunctional by her medical practitioner, but her pain, like that of many women, was in actuality due to a lack of arousal, which is the most frequent cause leading to painful intercourse. It's not just young, sexually inexperienced women who report dyspareunia from low arousal. I hear the same complaint from many married women who were easily responsive earlier in their relationships. Now they have accepted or even directed a lovemaking pattern geared toward their male partner. Women often tell me they are frustrated with themselves for taking so long. "Taking so long compared to whom?" I ask. Compared to their husbands? Yes, it takes her twenty to forty minutes longer

for the experience to be pleasurable and orgasmic. This is completely normal. Women's bodies demand lovemaking to be long
enough for us to relate emotionally and to feel good. Quick and
simple rutting often ends up hurting.

With enough sexual stimulation and turn-on, the vagina normally lengthens and balloons open slightly at its upper end. The
uterus lifts to leave a longer vaginal pocket to receive a man's
penis. Without proper physical excitement, intercourse can also
hurt deep within the vagina. Your partner's penis could be inad-
vertently hitting your cervix. This can be very painful! Tilting the
angle of the pelvis upward with a flat pillow under the woman's
hips for missionary intercourse often alleviates the problem. Deep
pain, though, may signify ovarian cysts or endometriosis and
should always be investigated by a gynecologist.

Three Stubborn Pain Problems

Physicians and sex therapists most often see women experiencing
one of three types of sexual pain problems: "the three V's." These
conditions can be more complicated than the above causes of
pain. Because they are not part of our daily vocabulary, I'll explain
a little about what they are:

- Vulvodynia means pain anywhere in the vulva. Pelvic pain
  specialists Andrew Goldstein, M.D.; Caroline Pukall, Ph.D.;
  and Irwin Goldstein, M.D., authors of *When Sex Hurts: A
  Woman's Guide to Banishing Sexual Pain*, write, "You're likely to
  be diagnosed with vulvodynia when your doctor can't find
  anything else wrong with you, but you still have pain in

your vulvar area." Often the pain is constant, but some of my patients have it only with sexual excitement. I've talked to women who cannot stand their clitoris being touched once aroused. Unbearable sensitivity will sometimes occur when they sit with their legs crossed. Simply wearing underwear can cause women to experience continuous burning sensations. The chronic pain is potentially neurogenic (stemming from nerve damage or within the nerves). Oral tricyclic antidepressants like nortriptyline or gabapentin, which are used to treat diabetic neuropathy, sometimes bring relief. Sometimes vulvadynia involves the lower muscles that support the vagina (levator ani muscles) due to tension or pain anxiety. When musculature problems cause or complicate vulvadynia, physical therapy will be necessary to treat the problem.

- Vestibulodynia (sometimes called vestibulitis) is pain at the entrance of the vagina and is a subtype of vulvodynia. Though sometimes demarcated by an inflamed red margin, the skin may appear normal and the diagnosis must be made based on careful analysis of the painful symptoms. Intercourse is frequently described as "burning." Usually the vaginal opening hurts when touched during sexual intercourse, or even when touched randomly during a physician exam with a Q-tip. But not always. Other patterns include pain only upon arousal. Frequently, the lower crescent of the vaginal opening has the most sensitivity. New research suggests the use of birth control pills as a potential cause of this condition in young women.[4] If a woman has always had it, it may be a congenital birth defect. Or her hymenal ring may need to be expanded surgically. Often it develops without any apparent reason and women wonder what is wrong with them to make sex hurt so much. Treatment often begins by using topical medications like lidocaine (used to rest the sensitized pain nerves) compounded with estrogen or testosterone for deeper healing of the cells. Oral medications may be used. As a last resort, surgery to remove the painful margins may be required and often has excellent results. Again, the levator ani muscles may be tense and add to the pain. Physical therapy is then part of the treatment.

• Vaginismus means a woman's vaginal muscles contract in spasms severe enough to prevent sexual penetration. Gynecological exams are difficult or impossible. A vaginismus sufferer may be unable to use a tampon. Secondary vaginismus results from surface tissue pain such as vestibulodynia when women, wary of pending discomfort, unconsciously clench their vaginal muscles to prevent pain. Vaginismus as a primary condition always requires psychotherapy and is due to some unconscious level of anxiety. Sex therapy and a woman's health physical therapist are helpful in resolving this condition. Ongoing trials are exploring the use of Botox to stop the reflex spasms for willing and motivated patients.

Unconsummated Marriage

Jennifer, thirty-two, was a late bloomer and her marriage of two years was unconsummated. As a premarital couple, she and her husband had lightly experimented with sexual touching and in no way anticipated such difficulties. Their wedding night had been filled with considerable trauma and tears when her husband, Theo, had been unable to penetrate her during their first full sexual experience. With her encouragement and without tremendous sexual experience himself, her husband had made repeated attempts, ending with Jennifer feeling bruised in her vulva and like a failure in her mind.

Waiting for two years before seeking treatment was a clue to me that there might be anxiety for both partners about sexual intimacy. A woman with vaginismus frequently describes her husband as kind and careful not to pressure her. Unfortunately, primary vaginismus is rooted in deep anxiety, and without a counterbalance from her partner's desire to make progress, a woman can remain baffled by the condition but frequently unmotivated to solve it. Jennifer and Theo could have at least resumed sexual touches that felt good or proceeded to orgasm, but they had begun living more like roommates than lovers.

When I evaluated Jennifer's sexual history, I did find issues familiar to my other vaginismus clients. She had had one successful but painful gynecological exam before marriage, and her doctor had reassured her that it hurt only because she was a virgin. He said her anatomy was normal and did not anticipate that she would have any problems with sex. Jennifer had never used tampons simply because she found the thought of them gross. She also used a washcloth to clean herself and could not remember masturbating, or experimentally examining or touching her genitals. Her vulva was not fully integrated as something that belonged to herself.

She had rigid beliefs about sexuality—especially that it was to be reserved for marriage. She told me about a time of "rebellion" in her late teens when she had experimented with alcohol and boys. I asked her about potential guilty feelings over these years and she affirmed that it made her feel terrible that her husband was not the first man to touch her intimately even though she had not previously had intercourse.

Suspiciously, a male friend of her family's had been her caretaker when he was temporarily out of work and Jennifer was about four or five. Knowing him most of her life, she thought of him as a fairly unstable character even now, occasionally drunk at her family's gatherings and often inappropriate in his jokes and innuendos. Her moral rigidity seemed to spring reactively from a childhood background of neglect and chaos.

We've talked about how vaginal pain can come from physical problems and how stress, anxiety, and our state of mind can make it worse. Primary vaginismus has psychological roots. Fear of being hurt upon penetration, moral rigidity, previous and perhaps unremembered sexual trauma, and/or deep anxiety about the self can cause the musculature at the opening of the vagina to be as impenetrable as a brick wall. It would take no less than two years to help Jennifer come to a point of psychological healing and readiness to tackle the actual symptoms of vaginismus. Her husband, Theo, likewise, had to resolve his anxiety about aggression and doubt over deserving good things from life.

Once a woman is ready in her mind, she can begin progressive behavioral steps toward full penetration. First, she has to integrate her vulva into her body image and become comfortable with touching herself. All penetration and attempted penetration should be accompanied by good artificial lubrication. I suggested that she insert her own fingers into her vagina. In this way, she remains totally in control and has the perfect biofeedback mechanism of touching and being touched at the same moment. Manufactured vaginal dilators, though, may also be used if they reduce anxiety. Glass dilators (Pyrex) will warm to the woman's body temperature. While a woman might have to tolerate some anxiety and a bit of discomfort, each step or half step should be designed to avoid pain. Once digital penetration is no longer painful and she feels comfortable giving up a measure of control, a woman's partner can be involved in the process. He also uses his fingers for progressive penetration during her sexual arousal. Concurrently, if the woman is anorgasmic, having her first orgasm can be an important step in learning to release intimate control in the presence of her husband. By the time he can penetrate her with three fingers and she experiences no discomfort, they are ready to try intercourse again. Many of my clients also are helped by physical therapy after they work through their psychological issues and are ready for behavioral steps.

Sex Suddenly Started to Hurt

Mandy wore her naturally graying hair long. She seemed caught in the 1960s in her midcalf shift, but she was troubled by the very present pain of vestibulodynia. The condition had come on suddenly and mysteriously. One day she felt a slight burning during penetration, and from that day forward, the pain increased. She hadn't felt normal since then. She didn't want to have sex again because it hurt.

Mandy and her husband, Vern, lived on a few acres and grew some of their own vegetables, trying to live as self-sufficiently as possible. They kept bees for honey, and Mandy would catch the hives on her own. Using a bucket, she'd capture the queen and scoop the hive, transferring the bees to their waiting home, where she fed them sugar water in winter and supplied them with fresh water in summer. She remarked to me that the occasional sting was nowhere near as painful as her continuous vaginal problems. Mandy and Vern spent evenings listening to jazz and talking. They didn't watch television. Their relationship seemed simple and sweet. With few expectations from life, Vern felt nonetheless hurt and depressed because he had lost his easy sexual partner as well as his traveling companion. Before Mandy's vulva condition made it too painful, they took extensive trips on their Harleys. These were people who didn't trust the system much and had already been let down. My office was the last place they expected to land.

Unfortunately, Mandy had some medical treatment that had made things worse. Because the causes of vestibulodynia are so complex, women often go through multiple treatments before finding what works. At first, she thought it was yeast. The diagnosis was incorrect and the over-the-counter yeast treatments caused an allergic reaction in her sensitive tissue. Then her first doctor prescribed steroid cream, which had turned her vulva bright red. While originally there had been pain during and immediately after intercourse, now the pain seemed constant. She called the doctor about continuing the cream. Without a reexam, he insisted she keep using it and her raw vulva soon looked like hamburger meat. Small cuts and fissures rimmed her vagina. Steroid cream might work for the right diagnosis, but in this case the diagnosis was wrong. I referred her to a local pelvic pain specialist who prescribed a compounded prescription cream of estrogen and lidocaine that finally began to heal the damage. This specialist has an arsenal of ideas and works with women until the problem is solved. I knew Mandy was in good hands. Like many women, Mandy's problems had gotten worse because she had tried to keep up sexual intercourse on her better days, and the excruciating pain had left her tense and anxious.

If I'd met Vern on the street, I might have been intimidated by him. His imposing height, long hair, and leather biker wear contrasted with the polo shirts and seersucker suits that generally walk through my door. But when he began to describe his disappointment in life, I was drawn to this gentle man.

The couple's sexual and emotional life had been hurt by the physical problem. With a soft country cadence, Vern began, "Miss Laurie, there has never been a point in my life that I thought to be in a counseling office. But we have nowhere else to turn. After my first marriage, I was a broken man. Then I met Mandy. I don't know where I'd be without her. But she's begun to shun me. She won't let me touch her even if it isn't to begin sexual relations. She won't kiss me or lay in the bed with me. At first I even thought she was making up excuses. Our life is not turning out the way I'd hoped."

Mandy was depressed too. Because she and I had met in my office before Vern came to see me, I knew she felt as much despair as Vern did over their disintegrated sex life, though she seemed painfully shy when talking about sexual issues.

I asked him how much she had shared about her medical treatment and her conversations with me. He knew that the first cream had tortured her. He said that having seen Mandy's "painful privates," he wasn't some ogre who would expect her to have sex with him in that condition.

Sexual intercourse was out of the question for the short run.

With medical treatment under way, our goal was to get these two connected in ways that expressed physical love but that didn't hurt Mandy. I coached Mandy to talk to Vern, and she tried.

"I want to make Vern happy. When I see him becoming, ah . . . involved with what we're doing in our intimate time, I want to make him feel good. Sex is very important to Vern and I know his first wife refused him. I don't want to do that."

Vern, speaking from deep frustration, tossed out, "Woman, what do you take me for? Even before, the only reason I would go ahead is because you said it was okay. I don't want you to hurt."

Throughout their marriage, Mandy usually had orgasms through sexual intercourse. She was reserved about any other form of lovemaking, Vern told me. Unfortunately, the more he opened up, the more Mandy stiffened and turned away. She found it hard to speak, finally explaining that where she came from, no one had talked about sex and she'd never really felt comfortable doing so.

Mandy had a high school education and a great deal of common sense. Unfortunately, her sexual education was abysmal. She had absorbed angry, primitive, prohibitive messages about "things prostitutes did" from her mother. I was the first woman she had ever talked to about actual sexual acts and her experiences. As the pain eased, she was able to separate her early training from her life with Vern.

If she'd been less inhibited, Mandy might have talked with Vern earlier and arranged comfortable ways to maintain their connection sexually. Not knowing how to talk about it, she needed coaching to use her words to reassure Vern of her enjoyment of their life together. If Vern had not been so scarred from his first marriage, he might have been more resilient and led the way. Mandy had believed that "having sex" meant penis-in-vagina and that she was failing Vern because she didn't want the accompanying pain. We explored a new definition of sexual connection that included pleasure, touch, sensuality, orgasms, connecting, and holding. I talked to this down-to-earth woman about a form of lovemaking called Tantric sex that emphasizes the delay of orgasm, prolonged arousal, synchronized breathing, and the increase of soul connection between lovers.

The Healing Process

Three branches of professional help aid the healing process when pain has interrupted sex. First, you need a physician who listens and with whom you feel comfortable discussing sexuality. Pelvic pain specialists are often necessary when initial treatment doesn't help. Because I have so much hope that the majority of pain problems can be resolved or at least made considerably better, I highly stress that women aggressively manage their medical treatment and find experts who can help. Don't suffer.

However, some pain issues cannot be fixed through medical treatment alone or at all, and sometimes you need the second branch of the solution: a specially trained woman's health physical therapist who understands vaginal musculature in the pelvic floor. Her role is to teach you which muscles are tightening and how to bring the problem under conscious control. Sometimes, a PT may use deep pressure or vaginal massage, or suggest vibration to unlock tense, tight trigger points in the muscles. Partners may be invited into sessions to learn about vaginal rehabilitation once the vaginal tissue is healed. No woman is completely comfortable with a gynecological exam because of its intimate nature. As an experiment to ascertain the level of embarrassment I was asking women to endure, I went to a women's health physical health therapist myself and asked that I receive the same exam. I am no more comfortable than any other woman in the stirrups. But the professionalism of the therapist made me comfortable and my visit was highly informative. I felt more collaborator than patient.

Third, a sex therapist can help with the technical aspects of comfortable intercourse, as well as providing work-arounds so that the couple can be sexual even if in a limited way. Resolving psychological causes or contributions to the pain problems require psychotherapeutic help. With Vern and Mandy, for example, therapy helped provide a safe, more complete pattern of communicating about erotic needs during the healing period. It also helped Vern not to feel rejected.

As mentioned earlier, sometimes there are simple explanations for pain. Before going to the doctor, a woman can try the following simple steps to see if they bring relief. Bring the following list with you to your doctor's appointment to show the changes you have made to get better:

- Wear white cotton underwear, and use a second rinse cycle during laundering to reduce detergent residue.

- Stay chemical-free—no soaps, dyes, deodorants, bubble baths, shower gels, or douches. Use unscented tampons, pads, and toilet paper.

- Use a handheld showerhead to clean the vulva and remove soap film traces.

- Sleep without underwear.

- Neutralize oxalic acid with calcium citrate under physician's orders. Increase omega-3 fatty acids and/or vitamin E under doctor's orders.

- Keep a chart to see if irritation is tied to your menstrual cycle.

- Neutralize acidic vaginal discharge with a cup of baking soda in a shallow bath the week prior to your period.

- Track when and where the pain occurs: arousal, penetration, postcoitally, urination. Think of the vagina as a clock; at what hour does the pain hurt most? How long does it last?

- Note type of condom used and check for latex allergies. Test by switching to a polyurethane condom (not as effective against STDs, however).

- If pain is accompanied by frequent urinary tract infections, see an urogynocologist to rule out interstitial cystitis.

- Have a gynecologist evaluate the use of birth control pills or need for hormone therapy.

When Really Bad Stuff Happens

None of us can anticipate the curveballs that life throws us. Most of us will never have vulvar pain except during short recovery periods after childbirth or perhaps in the menopausal transition.

But for some women, pain and low libido can be a side effect of dealing with cancer.

Mallory, forty-eight, had been diagnosed with estrogen-receptor-positive breast cancer two years earlier when she first came to the center. After a double mastectomy, radiation, and chemotherapy, she was recovering and was currently cancer-free. Now she was on aromatase inhibitors, a newer medicine that blocked the enzymes' synthesis and reduced her overall levels of estrogen. The cancer treatments had diminished her sexual response, and she missed the vitality of sensations and lovemaking with her husband that used to make her feel most alive.

At her first session, she narrated her cancer history. Just one month after a routine breast exam at her regular gynecological appointment, she had discovered a small lump in her breast. Ignoring it for a month because she had just been examined, she finally called the doctor back for a recheck, mammogram, and eventual biopsy. She was terrified as she listened to the diagnosis, but then set out on her course for healing. Researching her condition led to second medical opinions before she settled on an aggressive treatment. She was healthy and robust and wanted to make sure the cancer was gone. The doctors offered a good prognosis. After a double mastectomy, she underwent painful breast reconstruction, and her husband stood by her. He reassured her that she was sexy and attractive, and she said his loving perspective had healed her insecurity.

The best predictor of a woman's recovered self-image after breast cancer is her husband's communication that she is still beautiful. It's the same with prostate cancer. When a wife continues to affirm her husband's virility, his recovery is more complete.

A couple's love and assurance have great power to heal each other.

"The treatment was hell," she told me. "I'm glad it's over. My family and church provided terrific support, though, and that helped us over the worst parts. I'm not even here because of my breasts. I do miss their sensitivity, but I feel like I've accepted this. Ever since the treatment, though, my vagina has been extremely dry and tight and intercourse has been really painful. I ache to make love to my husband. He has given me so much love through this ordeal."

Desire came from love in Mallory's case. She didn't feel it in her body and probably wouldn't given her circumstantial limitations. But she wanted help in finding ways to make love pain-free.

Mallory's oncologist had forbidden the use of hormone replacement, even vaginal estrogen cream. Her kind of cancer was estrogen-receptive-positive—fed by estrogen—and nobody wanted her to take any chances. Many times that decision changes when the quality of life is weighed against the small risk of local vaginal estrogen.[5] A small study of women survivors on tamoxifen (a medicine that blocks estrogen differently) showed no risk to mortality in breast cancer survivors using vaginal estrogen.[6]

Testosterone supplementation to increase desire was also out of the question because testosterone is broken down by the body into dangerous estrogen-related by-products. Unfortunately, Mallory's chemo had hurried menopause. Making love during her treatment had been too sad, reminding her of all the sweetness she stood to lose. Not to mention the fact that her panic over the cancer had made relaxing impossible. After a year, her vagina was now dry and smaller. "Vaginal atrophy," her doctor told her.

While Mallory said she no longer mourned her lost breasts, losing a breast or both breasts is an enormous blow to a woman's sexual self-esteem. Breasts are the most prominent visible marker of our femaleness. In our culture, where appearance has an extremely high value, we are breast-obsessed. Physically, even if there is reconstruction, all sensitivity is gone from the nipple and we lose a stimulating pathway to arousal. When loved ones tell breast cancer survivors not to worry about their lost breast and just be thankful to be alive, they short-circuit the natural process of grief that brings full recovery. Women need permission to grieve and rage and cry over the losses to their femininity and sexuality.

The lamentable thing about breast cancer is that mastectomy is only the first loss to sexual functioning. Lymphedema, swelling in the tissues due to the removal of lymph nodes, may reduce range of motion in a woman's arms. Holding one's lover or stretching languidly with arms overhead when making love can be difficult. Lower estrogen levels can decrease vaginal lubrication and expansion. Sexual desire may be impaired or utterly zapped by the instant menopause induced by chemo or by prophylactic oophorectomy (removal of ovaries). Hot flashes and night sweats can arrive prematurely without the aid of hormone therapy. Weight gain is typical because of the use of steroids during treatment. Fatigue may reduce a woman's ability to exercise or manage her weight, further reducing her feelings of control over her body and her self-esteem. And tired women rarely have much energy for sex. Many cancer patients are put on antidepressants to combat the anxiety, fear, and depression of having their lives threatened and completely interrupted. In Mallory's case, I felt it well worth the possible medication disruption to request a reevaluation of her antidepressant. Her physician did switch her SSRI from a sexually impairing type to a dopamine-increasing type that didn't have sexual side effects.

I asked Mallory if she or her husband needed the full length of her vagina to produce orgasms for him. In the past, she had had no problem accommodating his size, but no, she imagined he would have an orgasm if she could bear even half his length. She had never had orgasms with penetration anyway but had enjoyed the feelings of connection with him inside her. Partial penetration attempts were prescribed after Mallory followed some of the following suggestions.

Rehab Tips

Vaginal rehabilitation for Mallory and others in similar situations takes the following steps:

- Assessing and treating the vaginal tightness and atrophy through weekly appointments with a physical therapist trained in women's pelvic-floor health.

- Developing more control over pelvic muscles in treatment, learning to relax them.

- Resting for four to eight weeks from intercourse while stretching the vagina.

- Orgasming twice-weekly through clitoral stimulation to increase blood flow to the tissue either through partner stimulation, masturbation, or vibration.

- Using vibration as the easiest route to orgasm due to hormonally-impaired responsiveness.

- Keeping the vaginal environment moist with a water-based suppository product designed for proper Ph balance.

- Massaging the vulva tissue with a press-and-release technique to work vitamin E oil (for freshness use the capsules pricked with a pin) from the clitoris down to the perineum.

- Dilating the vaginal cavity progressively and systematically on a daily basis beginning with the woman's fingers but adding graduated dilators/dildos to increase potential vaginal width and length.

- Increasing vaso-congestion through the prescription use of sildenafil cream and other agents that cause dilation of the blood vessels (only under a doctor's supervision) to increase sensitivity to orgasm in clitoris and vulva.

- Lubricating with artificial silicone-based personal lubricants every time without fail when attempting intercourse.

- Creating a measuring guide for husband's penis to help him control the depth of his thrust. Purchase a "vaginal sleeve" (synthetic toy used for mimicking a vagina) and cut it into a donut shape to slip onto his penis marking appropriate place that correlates with a comfortable vaginal depth. Other penile rings may prove too tight and uncomfortable.[7]

- Stimulating the clitoris and vulva slowly and gently to increase arousal to the highest level prior to intercourse. Penetration should be tried just before she crests into orgasm to take advantage of maximum engorgement in case her tissues empty and become flaccid too quickly post-orgasm.

- Relaxing in multiple ways: visual, music, vibration, romantic atmosphere, massage, and/or wine.

- Alternating through sexual positions to find ones most comfortable and easiest for woman to control depth and speed.

- Practicing other ways to bring each other to orgasm: oral sex, penis between buttocks, manual stimulation, vibrator stimulation for both.

- Accepting that he may never be able to penetrate completely again and grieving the sexual losses.

It took Mallory eight months of daily stretching to be able to have pain-free partial intercourse. When she checked in with me, she said she'd realized that in order for her vaginal tissue to stay open, she would have to continue very regular sexual intercourse and stretching. Her orgasms were back, but she claimed that, compared to her precancer state, they were weaker, and only one in ten was more than "a molehill."

Sex took lots more work now. I tried to comfort her by telling her that the natural aging process alone would eventually require expending more effort, compared to the ease of youthful sexual response most take for granted. Mallory had been cheated out of the gradual hormonal decline of a natural menopause. As they age, all women experience a reduction of lubrication, and without regular intercourse, they risk vaginal atrophy. Mallory continued in treatment to see if we could isolate the factors that made some orgasms more powerful than others.

Treatments for sexual pain are as diverse and specific as the problems themselves. Many sexual pain problems can be completely resolved. One young woman came into treatment with vestibulodynia after several years of pain so acute that she rated it a ten on every point round her vaginal opening. Within weeks of medical treatment and therapeutic instruction, she identified only a pain level of two at two specific points. Most of her sexual experiences had been marred by pain, when proper help would have cured her.

Treating pain problems can be complex and lengthy. While some results aren't completely successful, there are often vast improvements. Left unattended to, pain during sex kills your libido and won't just go away on its own. Women fear that things will never get better and are tempted to give up. Anxious thoughts of having to suffer pain forever can even make it worse. No matter what level of pain, it is important to deal with it, and the quicker the better. Because most women in my practice find much relief through a combination of treatments available, I strongly urge you to take heart and take control of your genital health.

Help Yourself

1. Have you ever experienced discomfort during sexual stimulation or intercourse? Do you only have sexual intercourse when you are highly aroused?

2. List the steps you have taken to manage persistent pain or discomfort associated with your genitals or sexual activities.

3. What testing, medications, interventions have you tried? Which specialists have you consulted?

4. How has the pain problems interfered with your sexual relationship at this point?

CHAPTER FIFTEEN

Desperate Smoke Signals:
I Can't Stand the Way
We're Living

Often low libido represents failed intimacy in a relationship. When, over time, two people—for whatever reason—somehow lose their deepest bond, sexual contact frequently diminishes or can disappear altogether. The loss of affection can eat away at feelings of kindness and respect. Often the man's testosterone still pushes him to desire sexual release, but as one woman said, "I just can't do it with him when I feel so little connection."

My client load is filled with couples in stony marriages that they don't necessarily want to end. Each partner secretly (or not so secretly) thinks the other is to blame for their problems. He's too critical. She's too cold. He doesn't listen. She doesn't give. They judge their partner as selfish and their own actions as a justifiable reaction. Years of frustration and resentment have piled up between them.

Sex, if it happens at all, has become less frequent, less erotic, less renewing, and infinitely less satisfying. Avoiding sex helps them avoid the sadness of their lost relational vitality. But without the reparative function of lovemaking, the ordinary wear and tear of daily living continues to separate the couple further.[1]

A woman may experience her own body as so erotically unresponsive that she comes to believe she's just not a very sexual person. Sometimes she thinks the gulf between her and her mate is due to her intractably low libido. Other times she knows her sexual unavailability is a desperate smoke signal: "Help! I can't stand the way we're living."

She Says, He Says (or Doesn't)

Carrie and Patrick O'Conner were middle-aged and had been married "forever," according to them. He had dark curly hair with just a trace of gray and wore a short-sleeved shirt that was straining at the buttons. She was grayer and didn't wear any makeup to conceal the dark circles under her eyes. Three children had worn through their patience and finances, with some minor adolescent rebellion, college tuition, and a fair dose of shouting and arguing.

"Patrick doesn't talk much," began Carrie. He replied that he'd talk more if she would ever get interested in the bedroom. Both were clearly unhappy and seemed mildly depressed. They also made it clear that there were no third parties involved in their conflict.

Asked what a typical evening was like, Carrie volunteered, "I trudge home from teaching and usually make dinner after stopping by the grocery store because I'm never organized enough to make a meal plan for the week. Then Patrick comes home. He usually wolfs down the food and disappears up to his office without so much as two words. Our kids have their own activities and basically grab dinner on the run. We haven't sat down as a family since our oldest was in grade school."

Quickly contradicting her, Patrick added, "Moira"—looking my way—"that's our daughter, eats dinner with her most nights."

"Yes, Moira is my sweet girl and our youngest." Carrie brightened only momentarily. "I don't really understand the boys. I feel like once they became teenagers, they were unrecognizable to me."

A child's coming-of-age is a difficult stage for many families. The O'Conners hadn't resolved the boys' need for independence with much peace. Carrie felt rejected and Patrick felt out of control.

I asked Patrick what he did in his home office. "I try to finish the work that is never done," he answered a tad defensively.

When I mentioned how joyless and stressed their existence sounded, they nodded.

I needed to know what the family looked like at their worst. Carrie, again, was the first to tell. "Patrick is incredibly angry. He and the boys have even had some physical fights. Our oldest won't come home when Patrick's home anymore. I travel up to his college if I want to see him. But he's as silent as his dad, so I end up hurt when I attempt to reach out to him. I'm here because we are splintering apart."

Patrick was quiet after her report, but I was getting the picture. I asked him why he was here, and he answered plainly, "I'm here because you're a sex therapist and I want to have more sex with my wife."

Their world broke down to arguments or silence. Family rituals and traditions had petered out. The only connection in the family I could ascertain was between Carrie and her daughter. They probably looked like anybody else to their neighbors. They kept their lawn mowed and cars washed. The kids were respectful to folks outside the family. It's hard to imagine all the sadness that really goes on inside people's homes and inner worlds.

Hoping to find a point of alignment with Patrick, I said that sex was certainly important for maintaining the connection in a marriage, and I asked him to tell me what happened between the two of them sexually.

"Not much."

Pushing him to elaborate would automatically seem as though I were siding with Carrie against this reticent man. I knew that many men boil down their anguish at a multitude of family and couple problems into one central complaint: no sex. It can be hard for their wives to understand how love can be spelled so completely and simply with three letters, S-E-X. A woman can feel used rather than understanding that sex is the way her husband connects.

I asked Carrie to fill in the blanks with her side of the story. "We have sex occasionally, but I admit, he's right—not often. Maybe my being perimenopausal has something to do with it. But I can't jump into bed with someone who I haven't had even one meaningful conversation with in weeks and weeks. He thinks I withhold from him, but all he seems to want is my body. Rutting with another body is not really my idea of a good time in bed. He doesn't care what's going on with me, and he didn't even ask what I talked about with our older son when I last saw him. The way he treats Sean leaves me cold inside."

Without laying a hand on her, Patrick's treatment of their child had left Carrie bruised. I knew that Patrick would relay hurts of his own in the sessions to come. Carrie's repeated references to the problem between her husband and older son told me it was probably the central reason she had closed off her heart and body. I didn't believe she was consciously denying him pleasure. But their romantic tie had been severed in her mind because of this injury to the family. Furthermore, as I've said before, most women need something soulful, some kind of emotional connection, to feel sexual. But the lack of time they spent together and their habit of relating only when absolutely necessary was hardly conducive to a firm bond.

I scheduled three sessions alone with each of them before having another joint appointment, hoping that without Carrie there, Patrick might be more forthcoming. He had the equanimity to accept my recommendations. I also hoped to comfort Carrie and help her feel stronger for the fight ahead.

Believing in Ghosts

By middle marriage, say after a decade or two, families have evolved into complex layered relationships—spouses with each other, each child with each parent, and children with one another. Personal hurts each partner has suffered in the past have impacted the marriage and the way they raised their children. Now the children are active parties, complicating things further. Crises of various sorts—economic setbacks, illness, death, taking care of both children and parents—have taken their toll on the union.

In her session, Carrie told me about the beginning of their relationship. "Patrick was a reckless, bad-boy Irishman and I was crazy about him! Once he drove his car up the steps of my dorm and honked and hollered for me to go out with him."

Their troubles began early, though. "I converted to Catholicism for him," she continued. "Not that he was very religious, but I think he wanted his father's approval. His parents didn't even come to our wedding. His dad just couldn't move on and forgive Patrick for the trouble in his adolescence and his mom always kowtowed to Patrick Sr. She might have sent a gift, I don't know. We didn't have sex that night 'cause Patrick passed out drunk. I think because he was so disappointed. At the time I didn't realize it was about his parents and thought he was upset with me, so I spent my wedding night crying alone and watching reruns.

"Years later, his mom usually remembered the children's birthdays with cards, but even though his parents didn't live that far away, they never came to see the kids. I suppose I couldn't forgive them for not loving my babies. Then my father didn't like Patrick; he thought I could do better. And Patrick hated him. So we didn't get off on the right foot with my side of the family either."

As we saw with Karen and Simon in chapter one a honeymoon misunderstanding was still hurtful to Carrie after years of marriage. The disapproval of their families, and the distance the latter maintained, left her and Patrick without their parents' wisdom or experience to help survive early marriage or early parenthood. Whether they could have helped the young couple is questionable, but the lack of family support during those years was another stressor. Furthermore, both partners carried blueprints in their heads that adulthood was incompatible with continuing support from one's own parents. To be an independent adult meant a total shutout from a relationship with your parents.

When Patrick scorned using birth control after their third child, Carrie stopped having sex for fear of pregnancy. "Patrick was so angry with me that he withdrew and stopped touching me altogether. I felt controlled by him, but he blamed me and said I was controlling. It was like we were chasing our tails. Even now I'll reach out for his hand when we're walking and he won't squeeze back. I feel constantly rejected and he thinks I should want to have sex with him? I don't even know him anymore. There might be parts that I still love, but I absolutely hate him for what he's doing to the children. He's become his father."

I believe in ghosts. Not the spirits of dead people lingering in a house, but pale, vague resemblances of people who may still be living and are capable of disturbing us with unfinished business from our past. The O'Conners were being troubled by these flickering traces of their history. Like Hamlet and his father's ghost, we are mired in agendas sometimes not of our own choosing, some of us growing fretful and more depressed as the years go by. Again, analyzing families and past relationships makes us aware of the ghosts that disrupt our present connection. Harville Hendrix emphasizes that we "do not know the extent to which we continue to be influenced by . . . ghosts from each partner's past. Mothers, fathers, former lovers, best friends, coaches, and special teachers occupy the Between" of every partnership.[2] Psychologists like to call these ghosts objects and projections. Marriages are often haunted.

These ghost images from childhood are based on memory, but also on our childlike—that is, partial and particular—interpretation of what actually happened back then. Hence brothers and sisters can have completely different views of their family because of their unique personalities, birth order, and vulnerabilities. All the good that comes from our background is used to make us strong. But the bad stuff from our past hangs around making mischief and malevolence, waiting to be released should we ever concentrate, see it, and attempt to exorcise it. The past governs our feelings about how close to be and how much independence we need for safety in our intimate relationships. And unfortunately, sometimes we see a familiar and scary apparition on our partner's face, and we react not to our partner but instead to the ghost of family past.

Banishing the Ghosts

Understanding the family that we came from doesn't offer us excuses for dysfunctional behavior. Our parents are not fully to blame for our problems. The ghosts might be aspects of them, but they are not them in totality. Not to mention that our parents have often outgrown who they were in their early and middle marriage, which is why I caution people from running home and screaming at their folks. But understanding the ghosts helps us understand why we feel so frightened (sad, angry, disrespected, abandoned, etc.) in a particular situation. We can see why we react in old and perhaps inappropriate ways. We have choices when we are able to think instead of being possessed by these old spirits.

For instance, when you turn down sex, your husband may feel ghosts coming out of the woodwork: the child that lay in a wet uncomfortable diaper too long, the mother who was too busy to hug him while nursing a sibling, a father whose embrace was stiff and awkward, his lonely teenage years with too little family affection. His disappointment is due in some part to your actual turn-down, but the rejection can also unconsciously trigger a reaction related to all the ways he didn't get love that he needed. Internal translation: no one will ever meet my physical needs and I must be bad for having these needs. His disappointment turns into despondency and shame. It might be tempting to say, "Oh, grow up—I'm not your mother!" But then when he pouts for the rest of the evening, you see a specter of one of your parents ignoring you. You remember your mother's silent treatment or your father running roughshod over your wishes. And on it goes.

I knew simply assigning homework would not fix the O'Conners. Date nights, family dinners, romantic getaways, communication exercises would all gleefully be sabotaged by the ghouls in their heads. Some partners, those who come from more comforting childhoods, are able to make use of straightforward suggestions without as much ghostly interference. But these people had more nurturance in the first place and came into marriage stronger and more whole. They can use tools, develop cognitive strategies, and learn to generate solutions to their problems. Neither Patrick nor Carrie had come from that type of family, as evidenced by the chaos and trouble they were having relating to their children. They needed counseling that was focused on building empathy, not simply communication tools. Their lives were crippled by angry, rageful, depriving, and controlling situations from their pasts. I wasn't sure what had happened between

Patrick and his elder son, Sean, but I knew for certain that ghosts were acting up.

Sexual healing for couples in this stage takes more than a bag of tricks. Families operate as an interrelated system. When the system is unhealthy, all parts of it reinforce dysfunction to some degree, either by direct action or by passivity. No one is completely to blame; nor is anyone completely innocent. Nevertheless, I felt sure the O'Conner family could find a more positive direction, where relationship and sexual love would heal their loneliness and cut-off feelings. A first step they could take toward correcting their inaccurate perceptions was to learn to contain their own judgments when listening.

Playing the Triangle

In his session with me, Patrick explained what had gone wrong with Sean.

"He's a smart kid, but he's so damn sensitive and whiny. I have to push him just to get him to move in any direction. Like Carrie told you, I did clobber him one time when he got smart with me. She protects him and just makes it worse. He's tied to her apron strings, whining to her all the time about his 'problems,' and she coddles him, listening to all his bellyaching. I want the kid to grow up and be a man, and he's never gonna do it with his mama babying him. For crying out loud, he hasn't declared a major and he's a junior. He'll never fuckin' graduate, and I'm gonna be stuck with the bill."

Listening, understanding, sensitivity, and interpersonal connection—Patrick denigrated them all. These were the very attributes that Carrie wanted in him so she could feel connected. Patrick was a tough guy; his own struggles growing up had left him cynical and crass.

I wondered about the boy-Patrick whom Carrie remembered as likable and passionate. In order to feel some sympathy for Patrick, Carrie (and I) would need to make the effort to see the more vulnerable person inside, someone who felt wounded and was drawing a protective shell around himself.

Early imprints from our first experience in a relationship of three—mother, father, baby—cause fragile places in our adult families. I wondered about the jealous ghosts that might be threatened by Sean's early closeness with Carrie. Was Patrick the odd man out in the relationship between mother and baby, feeling hurt and shoved aside? Had he wished to be closer to his own mother, and now envied what Sean had with Carrie? I knew that Patrick would instantly dismiss my suggestions as "full of crap" if I broached them directly, so I kept my mouth shut. But I did ask about his family of origin and he humored me.

"My own dad was a man's man. He didn't take shit from anyone. We fought some, so I got outta the house and was working by the time I was fifteen. I didn't come back, not even on holidays."

What must have sprung from deep pain over his ruptured relationship with his father was remembered by Patrick now in a way that sounded akin to respect. I asked Patrick how he'd feel to have his sons on their own at fifteen.

"Hell no, I don't want that. I'm working so it can be easier for them. But I don't want them to fuck around for the rest of their lives either. And I'd like a little appreciation for how easy they've got it."

Moving the conversation back in time, I discovered some of

what I'd worried about. Patrick's mother had been a mousy woman. She and his father had quarreled incessantly over little things. She gave in most of the time. Patrick didn't think they had had much sex, or at least he couldn't imagine it. His mother hadn't put up a fight when he left home, but that was because, he said, "I was really a rotten kid."

Who told him he was rotten? "My father, my teachers. Not my mother, but she was outvoted." As plain as day, I could see the story being reenacted with his son Sean. It's funny, but I always expect clients to hear themselves and be startled awake by the obvious repetition of themes. But we can be deaf to our own story, and only with the empathic ears of another can we begin to hear it. Patrick had fortunately married a woman with some of the nurturing aspects of his mother. Carrie's perceived sexual dullness, though, was also reminiscent of Mom.

Ah, there he was—the vulnerable Patrick I could (and came to) sympathize with—a troubled youth whose mother hadn't fought hard enough for him to stay in the family home and whose angry father had banished him. With clients and partners, sometimes seeing through to what might have been gives us the love we need to care for the shell that's left. Love that imagines the best in someone is a transforming force. Though, of course, that's easier for a therapist to feel than for a partner who depends on that other person to meet her needs.

I knew Patrick wouldn't like it if I felt sorry for him. But good therapy serves to show people how their own story can be incongruent with their spoken values. Patrick didn't want his own boys to experience the early independence he had known, but like his dad, he was pushing Sean out with his criticism and anger. The ghost on Sean's face was Patrick's own anxiety, dependence, and fear of the future. He was afraid of Sean's sensitivity because his own father had trampled his. Patrick thought that denying feelings and fears was necessary to becoming a man. Using his own rather distorted logic, he was trying to help Sean transition into adulthood.

Carrie, on the other hand, needed to stand up to Patrick where Sean was concerned. In my sessions with her, I encouraged her to follow her natural instincts in this direction for two reasons. First, it would provide a different ending for Sean than Patrick's story in his family of origin. Here, mother defends son and hopefully the tale ends with the reconciliation of father and son. Second, she couldn't be sexual with Patrick while this family wound remained gaping. At the least she would feel stronger and more powerful if she could make this reconciliation happen. The mousy mother of Patrick's past wouldn't be so mousy, and Patrick's respect for Carrie would go up. Sometimes, respect is a better target to shoot for than connection or understanding.

Broken Hearts

At the next joint session, Carrie energetically opened by announcing to Patrick, "Laurie told me that I shouldn't have sex with you until you see a therapist with Sean."

Looking at her, Patrick replied, "I guess you two women have it all figured out, don't you?"

Anxious about the effect this misinterpretation would have on Patrick, I asked Carrie as mildly as I could, "Is that the way you heard what we talked about?"

Carrie looked confused and defensive. "Yes, I heard you say I probably wouldn't want to have sex until I felt better about Patrick and Sean." Her glance spoke volumes. *Did I do it wrong? Why isn't this working the way you said it would?*

Trying to agree with and contradict her all at once, I said, "And I do think your desire is wrapped up in this conflict."

Patrick looked at me for the first time in the session. With some relief, he bit back a little at Carrie. "See, Carrie does that to me too. She twists my words. I don't know what she's told you, but she stopped being interested in sex with me long before I had it out with Sean."

Relieved, I hoped our three private sessions of trust building would hold. "Patrick, can you tell me what you felt just now when Carrie started us off?" He had already told me that he often felt criticized and attacked by Carrie, but I hoped to defuse any bad feelings from this encounter by directly asking about it.

"What did I feel when she said you had ganged up on me? Mad." He said this with a fair degree of calmness. By now, I knew Patrick felt anger in response to every emotionally charged circumstance. Feeling angry gives us a sense of energy, whereas feeling hurt, sad, lonely, or out of control can make us feel impotent. Patrick only allowed himself to feel or identify the hottest emotions because digging deeper would be more painful. People shrink in grief. Depression parks us on the couch. Hurt feels humiliating. Unfortunately, Patrick's inability to react with anything besides anger made his family afraid of him. I commented that it was a wonder he didn't feel despair.

Not realizing that Patrick was talking about his emotions rather than simply being overwhelmed by them, Carrie picked up the argument defensively as if the issue hadn't been settled. "We didn't gang up on you. My sessions were all about what I've done wrong. I've harped at you about what you've done wrong instead of asking directly for what I need."

When a marriage has broken down, couples bicker almost out of habit. Intensity substitutes for intimacy. In an odd way, arguing is the connection. While both partners may long for more listening, gentle conversation, affection, and sex, those acts shorten the distance between them, as we've discussed earlier. Distancers, anxious about closeness, afraid of being subsumed, strenuously avoid tenderness. Pursuers, not wanting false hope, give up on wishes for warmth. They have forgotten the original aim of resolving a particular problem. It's kind of like children who need attention. Even bad attention is better than nothing. Each spouse stops listening to what the other is saying because both are too busy formulating counterarguments in their heads. Carrie was so caught in their old ways of doing things that she didn't hear how the tenor of Patrick's statement was new and reflected his growing understanding of himself.

Carrie was correct, if defensive, about my focus in each of their individual sessions. While wanting to hear a couple's complaints and hurt feelings, I usually keep the conversation geared toward how their own actions keep in motion the very dynamic they don't like. If we can identify even a tiny part of a problem that we are responsible for, we suddenly have power to change the interrelated parts of the problem. Clients can't see or predict how their small changes will reverberate through their family and often result in big changes.

"Sean is absolutely beside himself that his father won't talk to him anymore," Carrie continued. "I think he's forgiven Patrick, but Patrick won't forgive himself. This semester, Sean is doing so poorly in school, and I think it's because he's depressed." In a stronger voice, she added, "You can be as critical of him as you want, Patrick, but you're going to have to keep it to yourself. I'm expecting you to do something to make this better. I will have all my children together this Christmas even if it means you won't be there."

I could have applauded Carrie for her firm stance. She needed to win an argument and be taken seriously. Otherwise, she'd continue feeling too dominated by Patrick to freely participate in sex. But I knew Patrick wasn't going to like her tone. I knew that he would balk at her insistence. And he did. First he tried bullying.

"If you think I'll be anywhere but my own home at Christmas, you'd better think again, Carrie."

"Then we'll go somewhere else, Patrick, but the children and I will be together." Carrie had guts after all. She looked at me. "He's going to make us end up like his parents, with none of the kids coming around to see them."

Back and forth the argument went. He'd seen his mother after his old man had died, he said, so Carrie didn't know what she was talking about. He's always so literal, she said. She's always critical, he said.

With her serious threat to leave him at the holidays, Carrie alternated in Patrick's mind between the ghost of his mother who let him go and the ghost of his critical father who told him he wasn't good enough. He was going to be without a family at Christmas—again.

Risking becoming a part of the fray, I suggested, "Patrick, I don't think Carrie is accusing you of being a bad son to your mother. She is saying she wants you to hold your tongue with Sean, though. And she wants more connection than your family seemed to have. What about you? Is this the way you want things

to be between you and Sean?" Perhaps his own desire for recon-
nection to Sean would offer the family a win-win solution.

Worn down a bit, Patrick made a last stand: "She needs to let
go of him. All the kid does is argue with me; he doesn't need me."

It's funny how sometimes we push someone away and believe
they pushed us. We can confuse the motives inside us with the
real players and the tricky ghosts.

"He does need you," I said firmly. "I think you feel stuck
about how to get the relationship back. You've agreed with me
that you're a bit depressed. I think this situation makes you sick at
heart, Patrick. What if your mother hadn't let go of you? What if
she had stood up for you? Your family of origin might have looked
radically different. Carrie seems to be trying to get the connection
that your family didn't have."

Patrick laughed humorlessly. "If she wants connection, what
about my needs for connection? I've been telling her for years, I
need connection in bed." He was diverting the conversation in the
direction that was crucial for him.

"Patrick, I do want connection with you, but I need emotional
connection before I'm ever going to feel like having sex again.
And every night you hole up in that office, sadder and sadder, it's
like our family is disintegrating. It's breaking my heart."

Soberly, he looked her in the eyes, his grizzly costume drop-
ping off. "You've held me off for years, Carrie. I don't have anything left to fight for us."

Carrie started to argue, but I stopped her. I wanted them both
to hear what they had meant without more words getting in
the way.

"Listen to what you've said," I urged. "You need each other.
You ache for each other. And both your hearts are broken."

Who'll Go First?

By becoming aware of this present moment of love and longing, perhaps Patrick and Carrie would be motivated to recommit to loving each other in the ways each craved.

It wouldn't be easy, because Patrick and Carrie had set up their dilemma to be unsolvable. He needed sex to feel connected and she needed emotional connection to want sex. Many times we feel that our immediate instinctual reaction to a problem is our only choice. I'm angry because you are angry. Or your partner does something insulting, hurtful, or stupid, and there seems to be only one option: get back at him. But to be autonomous in a relationship requires us to fix the ways we contribute to the problems regardless of the actions of the other.

This stalemate kept the O'Conners from each other. It kept them in a constant loop that maintained a familiar distance from each other. Twisting two problems together to form one issue made each of them dependent on the other for change—or so they thought. Parallel problem solving would require a commitment from them individually to grow in a direction that the other needed. Obviously a leap of faith is required to begin loving when the rewards might be months away. And seeds planted cannot grow if they are uprooted frequently in order to measure their progress. So each partner must commit to a season of change, with or without reciprocal effort from their spouse.

Carrie pursued emotionally and Patrick pursued sexually and vice versa with their distancing. They both wanted something from the other. Patrick needed to step toward his family and toward Carrie emotionally and she needed to step toward him sexually.

To untangle the two seemingly linked problems, I asked Carrie and Patrick to answer some questions:

- Is there any truth to your partner's complaint?

- If so, do you want your partner to feel differently and more content in the relationship?

- Do you feel that giving them what they need would cause positive growth for yourself?

For instance, if Carrie were to become more sexual now, in the short run, her increased eroticism might make her life happier and give her one form, albeit not her favorite, of connection. She would have to face up to her conflicted feelings about sex. Maybe she'd have to tell Patrick directly how she liked to be touched. Up to now, she'd been weak about directly communicating many things, so this would be one small way to strengthen herself as a person. She would have to face a myriad of assumptions about sex and women and marriage, including the examination of her parents' marriage. But in the long run, if this marriage failed, she'd have grown enough to bring a more erotic woman to her next relationship.

If Patrick were to learn to listen and become curious about Carrie's world, this skill would benefit him elsewhere—with his children, at his job, in other potential relationships.

Patrick's defensiveness stopped him from considering whether Carrie's criticisms were valid and whether listening might make his life better. He locked himself into a rebellious mode that made doing the opposite of her suggestions his only option. Real independence would come when he decided on the course of action whether it made her happy or not.

He had decided that women were a confounding mystery and had given up. I assured him that therapeutic coaching would help him understand his wife's needs and teach him more powerful ways to comfort her that didn't require omniscience. I also emphasized the need for his attention when he listened to Carrie. "Listening is more than just hearing," says Debra Fine in *The Fine Art of Small Talk*. "It's a level of involvement that goes beyond reciting the contents of the conversation." Fine describes a good listener as showing response, feeling connected, and being invested in the teller's story. I reassured Patrick that this kind of listening was more than enough to satisfy Carrie's need for connection and that if he practiced it he might feel less anxious about talking to her.

As treatment progressed, they were given practical tasks to perform. Carrie eventually demonstrated sexual love by looking for a moment when her mood was relatively open to initiating sex. Patrick was to turn his consideration to Carrie when he came home, after a brief time alone that he needed to settle himself. He was to ask about her day and give her attention for a short while. Cocktail-hour debrief was to be a complaint-free zone. For now, we designated the therapy hour as the only current time to discuss their frustration with the marriage.

The O'Conners had achieved a small breakthrough. They still had much more work to do before learning to reconnect and enjoy sexual intimacy fully. But the fog was lifting. For Patrick, sex was love. It wasn't all he needed, but it was the most tangible proof he could imagine. He was learning that he needed a family who stayed together emotionally even as the children left the home. Carrie needed to experience Patrick's love, presence, and friendship. She was grasping the truth that sex would lift the relationship out of the mundane.

Sean eventually came to a session with just his father. Without Carrie and her constant suggestions, Patrick was more able to see for himself how his son needed him. I affirmed his fatherly desire for Sean to have more discipline and drive. It was a different sort of love than motherly love—providing nurturing and empathy—but equally important for Sean. With a great deal of coaching, Sean shared his fear and grief about their fateful fight. While Patrick couldn't quite say he was sorry, by way of apology he did tell Sean about the fight he had with his own dad as a young man right when he left home. Carrie was enormously relieved that they were talking.

Lost in the Forest—Can't Find Home

Tragically, couples may wander in circles for years and years as if in a dense, dark forest, thinking they are impossibly lost. They contemplate divorce. They consider affairs. They fantasize being the relieved widow or widower. The path home may be steps away, but when a couple endures such despair for so long, they cannot believe anything or anyone can rescue them. Beginning the journey toward change takes tremendous courage. Even going through the tough work of marital therapy doesn't guarantee a happy marriage at the end, but it does challenge both partners to repair themselves. And that offers the couple a chance at happiness.

I've seen couples, even some who haven't had good sex in more years than they can count, come to terms with their difficulties, projections, and pain and be renewed sexually in wondrous, full, bodily resurrection. For most couples, there is a path to healing. Never an easy choice, the direction may be one they cannot take because resentment is too familiar and comforting a bedfellow. They may interminably wait for the other to go first, all the while withholding what their partner needs desperately. Stalemate.

But there is a way out of that seemingly hopeless place. As couples, we must accept that we can never know exactly our partner's motives or intentions. It's difficult to see through the nearly opaque screen of our own assumptions, histories, and limitations. We can change and that changes everything.

Help Yourself

1. Ask yourself if a repeating dynamic in your relationship might come from a ghost of family past. Write down the flickers of memory that seem related to a familiar dynamic between you and your partner.

2. List three positive and three negative qualities about your mother, father, and/or parental figures in your life. How are these qualities reflected in you and in your partner?

3. Discuss how deeper eroticism would benefit you regardless of whether your partner changes in ways you would like.

4. Practice listening with intention to both casual and intense arguments from your partner. Are the underlying issues the same?

CHAPTER SIXTEEN

Tough Conversations and Conflicts

Ned and Maria Holden entered my office like it was the stage in a theater. Hearty greetings, hand shakings, and big grins told me these folks were used to handling people. Indeed, as successful real estate agents and brokers, this dynamic duo made a good living from their image and people skills. In his mid-fifties, Ned was a handsome man. Muscular build, tanned face, taut jaw, he clearly worked at his appearance. Maria, mid-forties, dark shoulder-length hair, size six on the bottom and breasts well out of proportion, she was dressed in a boutique sarong skirt. Her fingers sported platinum and diamonds.

"Shall we call you 'Doctor'?" suggested Ned, flashing me a charming smile.

Shrinking a bit from their aggressive energy, I asked them to just call me Laurie. Whatever had brought this couple to see me,

I figured it was fairly difficult. People reaching a certain level of success aren't apt to bare their souls unless they are really hurting. Calculating that their bravado was masking quite a bit of anxiety, I let them introduce themselves.

Indeed, they presented their impressive social résumé—who they were, whom they knew. Within the first half of the session, I knew their net worth and a few other things that they probably thought they'd hidden. I knew that this was Ned's third marriage and he had grown kids he rarely saw. I knew they worried about money in spite of the appearance of abundance. I could see Maria's quiet acquiescence to the way Ned spun a story. Maria finally dropped the name of her gynecologist, who referred her to my practice.

Seizing the opportunity to guide the conversation toward the reasons they had come, I asked why the doctor made the referral. Smile frozen in place, Maria answered, "I told him that I've lost all desire . . . sexual desire. I'm not horny anymore."

Ned stayed jovial. "Yep, can't get milk from the cow now that I bought her."

I winced and looked at Maria to see how she had absorbed his comment, but unbelievably, she was still smiling. I asked them about their courtship.

"We've been married for eighteen months. I worked for Ned and helped him sell his last house," explained Maria.

"My wife, I mean, my ex-wife and I were having trouble at the time. Maria came into my life and just swept me away with her beauty and caring." Ned beamed toward Maria.

They had married as soon as his divorce was final. Blaming his previous marital failure on lack of sex, he vaguely threatened with, "My wife and I hadn't had sex for years by the time we di-

vorced. I will not stay in another marriage where that happens."
With these words, Ned sobered for the first time in our session.

"We had an affair," explained Maria. "I'd been divorced fairly
recently and Ned was everything I was looking for. He had a really
outgoing personality, which I need because social relationships
tire me out. His marriage was dead at the time, but we did get
together before they actually left each other. There were a few
ugly scenes with his former wife. She knew who I was and wasn't
terribly happy about us."

Sometimes an affair is used to find the energy to leave a marriage that is over, but for the rejected spouse, it's terribly difficult
and painful. And relationships that begin as affairs can face increased challenges regarding sexual trust. I decided to let the story
unfold as we went along. The Holdens had gotten together because of their sexual attraction and now Maria didn't feel anything.

"I think it was when I started gaining weight."

Noting her fit shape, I asked if she had lost the weight now.
Ned piped up. "No, she still carries it in her hips and thighs. It's
harder to see in that skirt. But I know she's working at it."

"Yes I am!" Maria averred. "It's very important to Ned that I
stay in shape."

"Right," said Ned. "We may be aging but that doesn't mean we
should go quietly into the night. Nothing about getting older is
attractive. I think we should do whatever we can to prevent the
inevitable. I'll go under the knife . . . whatever it takes!"

Ned looked like he might have already gone under the knife,
but I refrained from commenting. Thinking to myself that Maria
was only talking about the difference between fit and very fit, I
asked, "So, how did the weight gain impact your sexual desire?"

Maria looked at me like I was very dense. "He doesn't find me attractive anymore."

Ned explained, "Honey, it's not that I don't find you attractive; you're still cute. I just think you would be even more striking if you went to the gym more often." To me: "My first wife gained weight after she had the kids and never lost it again. I think it's disrespectful to your spouse to do that, don't you?"

People who have exacting standards of perfection are doomed to disappointment. If it's orderliness, the day will come when the laundry isn't put away. If it's moral perfection, your partner will tell some small lie and grievously create mistrust. If it's beauty, at some point we are past the knife's corrections.

It became clear that Ned's standards might be impossibly high when I considered how thin his wife already was. If the most important thing about one's spouse is her appearance, then deviating is viewed as a betrayal. Women already live in a cultural bind that asks them to look sexy but not to be too sexual. Perhaps a doll will look pretty and be compliant, but most men want an active partner. Sexual responsiveness to being desired is part of the normal female sexual pattern. But to be engaged sexually for a long-term commitment means also finding your own desire inside, not only as the reflection of a partner. Being sexual means having counter-demands. If you've married someone who sees you merely as decoration, it's dangerous to the arrangement to suddenly ask for longer foreplay or more cuddling and holding. Desire is fleeting in these relationships unless the couple does the work necessary to back it up. There is a common "narcissistic" myth for both genders that the most attractive person you can find will be the best sexual partner. False.

Making beauty the highest standard for finding happiness is a guarantee of failure. Every body ages. Women's breasts sag. Many have children and develop stretch marks. Their bodies may change permanently after childbirth. Either partner might get sick and face physical changes as a result. A happy marriage demands the ability to give versus gratifying self-centered desires.

I see so many women burdened by our culture's pressure to be impossibly slender. At first I pitied Maria. Many men would have absolutely gloried in her exotic loveliness just as she was. The classic exchange of a man's wealth for the beauty of a younger woman didn't make complete sense with Ned and Maria. First, she wasn't that much younger than he. Second, she could earn her own good living. As Ned was lacking some charm in my estimation, perhaps his greater wealth and good looks kept her in the relationship. I couldn't guess.

Mustering my neutrality, I levelly responded to Ned. "You really think it's important to stay fit for each other."

He nodded.

In an attempt to separate out Maria's feelings of genuine desire from her need to be sexually admired, I asked bluntly, "Okay, Maria, are you saying that Ned's desire for you to have thinner thighs means you don't feel horny anymore?"

"I don't like my thighs either," Maria said, deflecting the subject one more time. "It's not just Ned's desire but mine too. I am afraid that he'll be critical, but more than that I don't feel the excitement about sex that I did when we got together."

"When was the last time you felt horny?"

"I think I stopped feeling it when we moved in together."

Ned's frustration was becoming more evident. "I bought her dream house, and then after we moved in, my dream fell apart."

"What fell apart, Ned?"

"Maria stopped wanting sex for one, and she became critical too. Frankly, I feel tricked. I feel used," said Ned, this time with vehemence.

"I feel used too. All Ned wants me for is sex. He really isn't interested in what I think anymore or doing things together. He spends his time at the office and then I'm supposed to be powdered up and ready for him in the evening."

Each spouse felt cheated. Their boisterous demeanor fell away. Disillusioned couples often have what appears like copycat complaints. In Ned and Maria's case, there had been an implicit agreement. She was to adore him and be beautiful; he was to desire her and be attentive. They had struck a bargain that wouldn't hold up under real-life pressures. Whether this couple could deepen their relationship and connect with each other would mean long-term therapy. Unfortunately, pointing out too quickly the error of the foundation would probably do more harm than good. Waiting too long to help them gain more satisfaction in their relationship would make them give up on therapy. In our next few sessions, I settled for helping make explicit the feelings they had around attractiveness and sex.

"Ned, can you tell Maria what it feels like when she turns you down for sex?" I asked.

"Like she's denying me on purpose," he defined.

Sarcastically, Maria interrupted with a barrage of defensive counterpoints, "Would you be referring to last night when I was exhausted and you were scrambling under the covers to lift up my nightgown? God, I swear, you are like a greedy child after candy. It makes me feel like an object with no regard given for what I want."

"You know, sugar, after waiting a week for you to deem some moment perfect, I think I would call myself more desperate than greedy. Tired!? You spent the day with your sister!" Ned piled on.

As with so many couples embroiled in a power struggle, Maria and Ned weren't good at taking turns talking. Clear steps move a couple from struggle to empathy, where problem solving becomes possible. We must master the following progression of listening steps to move up the "good relationship" ladder. The listening pattern is: repeat, make sense, empathize.

- **Step one:** Repeat what our spouse has said without interpretation. No edge in our voice, no sarcasm. Paraphrase, not parrot. "You feel that I withhold sex."

- **Step two:** Make sense of what our spouse says from their viewpoint. We know our partner, we love him. We know the ways he gets hurt. Essentially, we must tell him that if I were in your shoes, I might think the same thing: "Certainly, we haven't had frequent sex lately." We must keep to ourselves the part inside that screams, "But you wouldn't think that at all if you understood ME!" There is time. We will have a turn. The minutes of discipline we exert to wait on our turn buys hours wasted on misunderstanding, confusion, and hurt.

- **Step three:** Empathize with your partner's feelings. Contrary to what most arguing spouses believe, agreement isn't necessary. If your spouse says they feel betrayed by an action, you know feeling betrayed feels bad. Telling your spouse that you understand they feel betrayed acknowledges their feelings without agreeing that you did anything to betray them. Not only is agreement or apology not necessary at this stage, but it actually gets in the way. Our partner just needs to be heard. Saying "I'm sorry I hurt you" without the other steps is a little like premature ejaculation. It might end the argument but probably won't be really satisfying for either party. Arguments are not about getting an apology. We need warmth, understanding, and connection.

Mirroring his complaint, "Well, I feel betrayed by you too," doesn't count. We must feel our partner from inside their heart. One brief moment of empathy is more powerful in building intimacy than any compromise. By the time we can use all three steps, we might not need therapy because we have expanded our capacity for closeness.

Maria could say, "If sex makes you feel loved and I don't seem to want to give it to you, I can imagine you would feel deprived and not cared about." She does not agree with: (a) she doesn't love him; (b) she is withholding purposely, or (c) she doesn't care. This is not agreement, admission, or acquiescence. Her empathic, careful restatement of his criticism is simply hearing him.

Getting the Message Across While Staying Connected

Similarly, it's very important to learn to speak in a way that generates the least amount of defense. The pattern for the sender of a complaint is: request, feelings, switch.

Step one: Request the change you want—directly.

For most people, the more concise the request, the greater the chance our partner has of remembering what it is you want in the first place when the emotions of the conflict take over. Let's look at a different couple for a moment. Kayla and Nora came to me early in their relationship to increase their sexual adjustment. In a fight, Kayla wanted to fix the problem. The longer Nora talked about things that made her unhappy, the more Kayla shut down. It made her feel helpless whenever she was the cause of Nora's anger. In the back of her mind, there was an echo of her mother screaming over some inconsequential chore that she had forgotten. Kayla would hear the first couple of sentences and then Nora seemed in a long tunnel far, far away. Her anxiety over intense emotions made her check out. Then she was so ashamed at her inability to respond quickly that she'd blow up or become absolutely silent. The thicker the emotion, the quicker were Nora's arguments. Kayla's verbal lockdown made her frantic and Nora would fill the empty space with more words. The distance between them grew further. Though as long as Kayla believed she had a shot at making Nora happy—even if it meant changing—she continued to listen. At least she tried to listen.

Sexually, Nora wanted more passion from Kayla. Always having more desire than Kayla, she felt burdened by being the sexual pursuer. She felt angry that after having asked for initiation, Kayla stayed passive, arguing that Nora didn't give her a chance to initiate. By pushing Kayla, I would only align myself with Nora. It was going to be a dicey conversation. I coached Nora to tell Kayla what passionate initiation would look like with very specific examples. I had her pick a time to tell Kayla—not when they were in bed, and not in the middle of any other argument. In the past she would wait until they were already angry to bring up other subjects that she was unhappy with. I explained how the anger was fueling her against her own anxiety over conflict. Unfortunately, fighting over several unrelated issues usually results in a tangled mess instead of resolution for any problem.

Nora was able to say, "Kayla, I want to make love when you are ready. I'll know that if you take the lead to get into bed. I'd love a seductive come-on. I'd like you to rub my back, eventually working your way down to my bottom. Then I'd like oral sex for a fair amount of time and even then I'd like to be touched some more with your fingers. I would love a luxurious thirty minutes of back-and-forth caressing."

Step two: Feelings are communicated not blame.

The complaint must be phrased in terms of emotions experienced rather than actions committed. The message "I feel unattractive to you when you don't initiate" was markedly different to Kayla than "You aren't a good lover."

Step three: Switch to listening.

Ask "What do you think about this situation?" or "Tell me what you like."

Knowing how difficult it is for any of us to hear criticism, we can immediately ask for our partner's experience of the situation. When we ask, we communicate that we know there are two sides to every story. Nora asked Kayla, "How do you feel about initiating?"

Hopefully our open attitude will reduce defensiveness and

our partner will first follow the listening steps before answering our gracious question.

Getting What We Want

When we learn to make requests directly and listen to complaints calmly, we smooth out our emotional connection. In turn, sexual connection stays steadier. Let's go back to Ned and Maria. In an ideal world, Ned could have phrased his grievance, "Maria, I want to make love three times a week" (request). "I'm feeling lonely and deprived with our current frequency of every other week" (feeling). "How do you feel about how often we make love?" (switch). Sure, there are plenty more details and examples of the problem. But in initial contact it's best to keep things short and to the point: request, feeling, switch (to listening mode). Much of my work during early therapy with couples is being a "launderer" of toxic dialogue. I help them say what they feel without damaging each other.

After several months of therapy, Maria came to see how much Ned needed the skin-on-skin contact of their lovemaking. She rose to the occasion and offered to have sex three times a week—twice in a quickielike fashion and once that she initiated when she felt desire. But Ned continued to complain about her small bodily imperfections. His criticisms served a purpose in keeping them apart sexually.

"Ned, when you criticize Maria, it dampens her sexual desire for you."

Ned defended. "Well, it's like you've created a monster. She's demanding sex all the time now . . . 'Honey, it's Thursday . . . are you up for it?' Now she wants me to specialize in the techniques you've taught us. I'm supposed to remember everything from one session to the next. Nothing is relaxed and spontaneous anymore."

Maria looked at me and then to Ned. "Can I tell her what's been happening?"

Ned was silent but glared at Maria angrily.

Maria braved on. "He can't get it up. It's happened a few times. Now he blames me for that too. He says I'm too demanding or too critical in bed. I'm only trying to direct him like you told me to." Turning to her husband, she continued: "I'm doing this all for you, y'know. You asked for more sex."

As soon as I heard her, I desperately wanted her to have said it differently. I wanted her to protect Ned's pride. Maybe "he's having a few problems with his erections." But I knew that Maria had been criticized relentlessly and unfairly. I remembered the comment about the cow and the milk.

I realized that much of Ned's fear of aging had been about his fear of impotence. Aging brings the loss of power in many ways, but for a man who has measured his worth by how well he can attract sexy women, erectile dysfunction is the kiss of death. In my experience, sexual dysfunction between partners is always managed together. Maria's low libido protected Ned from facing his erectile dysfunction. Ned's fear of impotence led him to criticize Maria so that she felt bad about her body and pulled away. His fear that she would discover his aging and reject him made him push away first.

Desperate to find some sympathy between them, I asked,

"Maria, how do you feel about Ned when his erection doesn't work?"

A bit of patience from her and my hope for this couple rallied. "I wouldn't feel so bad if he didn't just turn over and huff, like I'd done something wrong or was so unattractive that he couldn't respond."

In hopes of slowing down the pace of this argument, I clarified: "So it wouldn't be a big deal to you if it wasn't working and you decided to call it a night and just cuddle or have him please you."

"Men don't need to cuddle!" burst in Ned. "I swear to God, I've just about had it with the two of you women trying to understand what I need!"

"We're missing the point," I said slowly and carefully.

"Yes, you're fucking missing the point!" shouted Ned. "The fucking point is that my dick doesn't work with this bossy woman."

Seeing that he was on the verge of utter frustration, more firmly I reiterated, "Your dick only needs one boss—you."

"Yeah, my dick has one boss, thank you very much," he ended.

All three of us were silent for a few moments.

Ned composed himself. Still red in the face, he didn't like to lose his cool in public. To take some of the heat from the conversation, I had used simple reflective statements but avoided continuing his theme of blaming Maria. When someone is angry, hurt, or embarrassed, good listening responses have to be short and accurate. Ned wasn't ready for some sexual compromise. He wanted his virility to remain intact.

Therapy had been tough for this macho guy. Seeing a sex therapist was one concession, but a woman therapist made for two against one in his mind. Most of the time men find me unbiased, perhaps even a little on their side, since I'm almost always working to improve the sexual relationship. But Ned struggled with my gender even before this moment. He'd wondered if a woman could understand that men needed visual stimulation. He saw me on Maria's side when I stood up for her attractiveness. My communication coaching had helped smooth things out between them, but his concerns about aging and continued need for physical perfection in his partner had been driving the sexual wedge between them.

If progress was to be made, he'd have to fess up to some of the difficulty. And at this moment Ned already believed his manhood was in jeopardy. He'd been exposed before he was ready; he was vulnerable.

"So, you're just waiting for me to say that sometimes I can't even boss my dick around, aren't you?" Ned let loose with sarcasm.

"I figure that would be frustrating for you, Ned, if it were true." I mustered as much empathy as I thought he'd tolerate in this critical moment, hoping to help him preserve his dignity while shedding some light on his anxieties.

"God!" Ned wiped his hair back from across his forehead. "I'm telling you. Dick has a mind of his own. Sometimes he's as stubborn as I am."

I laughed; tension broke all through the room. Maria had enough good sense to stay quiet and not rub it in.

"Tough stuff for a man who's used to being the boss, huh?" I nudged.

"Humph!" Ned agreed.

He wasn't ready to talk about Viagra or the easy ways to fix his problem. For Ned, erectile dysfunction was a huge blow to his ego. As long as he could nag at Maria and keep her at arm's length, he didn't have to face the evidence of his growing older or his increasing shame. Her low desire protected him from his problems. He ensured her low desire by making her feel unattractive. His need for her to be extremely attractive was for proof that he could still capture the most desirable girl in the room.

Now that all this was out in the open, we could make real progress toward healing their sexual and relational rift. Once Ned began to believe that Maria actually loved him, he was able to let go of some of his perfectionism.

Maria did not instantly have high desire. But Ned's admission in this session went a long way toward his taking equal responsibility for the problem and it helped soothe her feeling that he blamed her for everything. She found a way to meet Ned's needs and her own with a frequency that amounted to about an hour a week. One lengthy session would last about forty-five minutes and she would have orgasms. The other one or two times, she would use a vibrator to get aroused or be on top and use a vibrator to climax. She told me she didn't want an orgasm every time but found the closeness enjoyable. The more she became available, the more Ned became satisfied with mutual experiences. As he became less uptight about his performance, he was able to both notice and appreciate how funny Maria was. His criticism had shut down her humor except in sarcasm.

Not willing to continue therapy for as long as I believed was necessary, Maria concluded our sessions with the comment, "Well, Dick's boss has decided that Maria's thighs might do as long as they wrap around him more often."

Talking about sexual needs and disappointments must be

handled with tact and care. In session, married people will some-times reflect that they just want to be able to say everything they really think or that they just want to be honest. Raw words, how-ever, about your partner's attractiveness, body, sexual technique, or desirability can be too hurtful to ever recover from. Maria was able to forgive Ned for his criticism after she realized it masked his insecurity, but not everyone can recover that successfully. Actu-ally, because we plan to stay a lifetime with our spouse, we must exercise the utmost discipline when we discuss intimacy and the changes we want.

Using the communication steps for listening to complaints and making requests feels awkward and cumbersome at first. Sometimes couples sabotage each other's efforts to change by ac-cusing their partner of "just doing what the therapist suggested." The detailed communication method takes longer than quick, sharp words. But the time saved from wrong assumptions and hurt feelings more than makes up for it. Knowing that it's normal to have disappointments at turning points in our sexual life can help us have the courage to talk. Then realizing that sexual prob-lems are circular dynamics rather than having a distinct begin-ning can help couples stop fighting over who is to blame. The goal becomes figuring out how each of them contributes to sexual pat-terns, and seeing that if these change, they would be happier.

Help Yourself

1. Name two changes you would like to see in your sexual life using less than eight words for each request.

2. Discuss which listening step is most difficult for you and why: repeat, make sense, or empathize.

3. Discuss what you think was, is, or might be important to you sexually in the following married life stages: engagement, honeymoon, first year of marriage, child-rearing years, midlife, and menopause.

CHAPTER SEVENTEEN

I Should Have Meant
More to Him: Affair Recovery

Nothing devastates a marriage like infidelity. While perhaps this desire problem is due more to the circumstances, a partner's affair can slam the heart and body closed. The injury you experience comes from the loss of being seen and valued by your intimate other. Up to now, your mate's commitment has deeply affirmed your being: I am because I am loved. Betrayed partners talk about being rocked to the depths of their soul with confusion, disorientation, and sometimes near-suicidal despair. For a while you have disappeared from your partner's mind and must struggle to exist in an unfamiliar world.

"How could I have meant so little to you?" asks a wife when an affair is newly discovered. And, indeed, at least for the short term, the couple's promises, their life together, and their children have mattered less than whatever personal needs prompted the affair.

When your mate gives to another what was deemed private, sacred, and special, you may feel unbearably violated. The wound strikes at the most vulnerable part of your relationship—your shared bodies and genitals. Even if the straying spouse doesn't ever say so, a primitive, accusing voice resounds in the betrayed party's head: "You weren't good enough in bed."

It's Not Just the Sex

In reality, as hard as it is to believe at the time, better sex is not the only reason people have affairs. While sex obviously plays a part, people frequently use affairs to redefine their existing relationship. There might be less painful ways to accomplish the same end, but it's not always easy for people to recognize the full range of their options.

I'm not excusing them, but I know that good people sometimes step outside their own moral frame when they feel desperate to change their lives. Perhaps they've truly struggled to change the marital sexual relationship only to be told by their partner that sex is not that important to them. Or the couple has fallen into a pattern of platonic companionship. Maybe the sexual relationship is consistent, yet emotional connection is missing. Occasionally a person seeks a new sexual relationship in order to be the uninhibited person that they believe the marriage will not tolerate. Sometimes one spouse so dominates the relationship that the other spouse sees an affair as offering the perfect rebellion.[1] It's not easy to accept such reasoning when the injury is so personal, but sometimes the affair has less to do with the relationship and more with one partner's emotions. And as with any complicated relational problem, there are frequently wider issues: job loss, illness, childbirth, children approaching their own sexual exploration, midlife crises, and aging.

Different types of affairs lead to different outcomes. Many people use the energy of an affair to end a marriage that they have long since left emotionally—it's an exit affair. Serial philandering is different from a one-night stand or an experimentation affair. Compulsive, nonpersonal sex on the Internet may threaten the family's financial well-being and both partners' spiritual integrity, while sex with prostitutes can endanger her very health. Believing one has fallen in love with another in a scarce month or two is different from a ten-year love affair. Once sex has been delegated to one person and love to another, a tough examination by both marital partners is necessary. Even then, there is difficult work ahead to regain trust and happiness.

Often, when their marriage and future are threatened with dissolution, both parties are frightened. I've worked with many couples who have had affairs, and I strongly believe that it doesn't have to mean the end of a marriage. If the spouses decide to work on the marriage, healing can emerge from this difficult crisis, and the relationship can grow stronger.

Two Years Later

Two years after her husband's affair, Frannie, in her mid-fifties, was still working to make sense of their salvaged relationship. They had seen a counselor when the affair was first discovered and both of them credited her with saving the marriage. Now Frannie was seeing me to save the marriage bed. She told me that she spent the first year trying to decide whether to keep her husband or to kick him out. Though she was still somewhat ambivalent, sex had resumed. But now Frannie struggled more than ever with her lack of desire.

Images of her unfaithful mate and his lover would go through her mind anytime Frannie and John began making love. "Then," she explained, "my imagination sort of runs away from me and I get a stomachache and sex is just over for me. I might urge him to go ahead and have his orgasm, but I'm totally turned off."

When she initially found out about the affair, Frannie had demanded details, and unfortunately, John had given them. Frannie believed that the only way she'd be able to trust him again was if she knew everything, including the erotic minutiae. But his explicit disclosure came when he was still angry and too close on the heels of her finding out. The images he painted traumatized her further; hence the flashbacks.

Transparency is indeed the first step in rebuilding trust if the couple decides to stay together. And it's understandable that curiosity, comparison, and insecurity would fuel the desire to know everything. It's essential that the straying spouse tell *how, where, when,* and *why.* Maybe describing *what* will be necessary too, but I believe only the rough outline should be given in the beginning, and the finer points, if they are told at all, be saved to share in the presence of a therapist. To rebuild trust, the involved spouse should offer up passwords on e-mail accounts, text, cell-phone access, and phone logs. For her own sake, the injured spouse should agree to set a limited daily time frame for a week or so to discuss the affair. Unlimited analyzing after a reasonable period of angry venting seems to deepen the anxiety of the injured party, and that usually leads to obsessions instead of constructive solutions.

John had opened his life to Frannie in an effort to reassure her about his commitment to honesty. He had cut off contact with the other woman after a conversation in which he expressed his regret to her as well. Frannie hadn't understood why he owed the other woman anything, but John had said, "Not explaining to her that I've decided to work on our marriage would only treat one more person badly. Whether you understand it or not, Frannie, I believe I do owe her that and it will close the door for all of us on that chapter." Frannie had reeled when she saw how many phone calls and points of contact they'd had over their six-month affair. Knowing him to be a deep person, she also knew John couldn't have just had a cheap, meaningless affair. There must have been an emotional connection, and that hurt even more.

"John believed he loved this girl, Laurie. That's what I find so hard to accept. He was good to me during that same time frame. How am I to know the difference now?"

I asked her if she and John believed they had understood why it happened.

With remarkable neutrality, she was able to summarize the problems that had led to the affair. "Yes, he entered therapy himself after it was over. And we saw our therapist weekly for quite a while. He says I tried to control him and that sex had gone flat early in the marriage. The therapist said his standing up to me about making the phone call to his girlfriend had been important. I'm still not so sure. I would have liked her to suffer some in the dark like I did. John was also struggling in a dead-end job and the woman gave him something very exciting to relieve the ennui of daily life. He's in a different position now and I've backed off on my demands, but sex is as flat as ever, maybe flatter. He says he knows I'm trying."

Had John told her what he loved about the other woman? "She listened to him and didn't demand anything, I suppose. No, I think he felt at ease talking to her, something he and I used to feel but didn't anymore."

Had he expressed remorse? Yes, he said he was sorry whenever Frannie spoke about the affair, and continued to be reassuring when the subject came up. After an affair, there are numerous reminders in daily life, including movies or TV shows in which it seems everyone is having affairs, or relevant dates will show up on the calendar (the date it began, the date she discovered it, etc.). When this happened, John would take Frannie's hand and squeeze it, confirming for her that he knew what she was thinking.

So although sex was still not so hot, and she worried about that, her husband seemed okay with the progress that was being made. Of course, it was harder for Frannie because of the additional hurdle about opening up to him sexually.

Five Steps to Recovery

To resolve an affair and revive a marriage, the following five steps need to be accomplished:

1. The involved spouse becomes transparent, a sharp about-face from the previous secrecy.

2. The involved spouse cuts off contact with the third party.

3. Both spouses accept responsibility for their contributions to the marital problems.

4. Remorse is expressed for causing hurt to the injured partner.

5. Intimacy is reestablished with deeper emotional and sexual bonds.

John and Frannie had completed all the steps except renewed intimacy. Sometimes the injured partner tries to monitor all aspects of her spouse's contacts. For a short time this might prove reassuring, especially if the mate is forthcoming (and I suggest that he be). But in the long run, vigilance is exhausting and doesn't serve to rebuild trust. The only path to real trust is through deeper intimacy. In intimacy—where both partners reveal their feelings, hopes, fears, dreams, and insecurities—connection underlies trust. Frannie wasn't sure they had that connection, which was why she remained anxious.

John had been struggling recently in his own therapy to be less passive in the marriage and to bring up problems openly. His pattern of listening had followed a typical male model of trying to fix Frannie's issues instead of understanding what she was feeling. He lacked the language for expressing his feelings and struggled with emotional intelligence. In some ways, his lack of self-knowledge had left him vulnerable to the affair. The woman had been younger and enamored of his more powerful position at work. After traveling together for work, they had started to debrief their days over cocktails. Her undivided attention had turned him on. He hadn't understood his feelings of exhilaration, nor had he articulated them to anyone else. Not really wanting to blow his cover by telling Frannie about his excited feelings, and not having the safety of male friends to listen to him, John had been unable to do anything but act on impulse. His lover had listened to his marital disappointments and together they had started on a risky path. John's admission that he was intimidated by and envious of Frannie's facility with emotional relationships with both their friends and their children was the most important breakthrough in the post-recovery period. He now realized that if he had been in touch with his needs and feelings, he might have brought issues up with Frannie and been more open to her needs and feelings as well.

Frannie revealed one more wrinkle that had hindered her sexual recovery. Their first therapist had asked John to describe the other woman. She apparently had larger breasts than Frannie, and the therapist had commented that perhaps John needed that erotic type to get excited. Frannie, naturally, felt insecure from that point forward. "What am I supposed to do, get a boob job?" she asked me. "I know in my head that couldn't be why he did it, and he's been repetitively reassuring about my body, but god, that still hurts."

While I respected the other therapist, this gaff had added insult to injury for Frannie. She had turned to someone for help and had been hurt. It was one more damaging comment that had to be healed.

First, I suggested we work on her base low libido, which had existed before the marriage, and then we'd deal with the intrusive images, and finally with this last hurtful comparison.

Heat It Up

Frannie's low libido had been due to many of the issues we've discussed in other chapters. Their routine had grown stale: bathe separately, go to bed, pull the sheets down, quick fondling, intercourse followed by a vibrator orgasm for her, and good night. She admitted that in the past, John had suggested some different things to try but mostly he had stopped this. He had wanted to tie her up and once asked her to put her finger in his anus. The first idea had scared her and the second shocked her, and she secretly wondered if he wasn't kinky or homosexual. Aggression, submission, domination, and variations on the theme flavor the fantasies of most people. When I explained that a man's anus had highly sensitive places and it had nothing to do with sexual orientation, Frannie sighed with relief. "I didn't think he was gay, but I'd never heard of any normal man wanting that."

Asked how many normal men she talked to regularly about their sexual desires, Frannie giggled and admitted that she had been a virgin at the time of their wedding and had certainly not talked with anyone else. Were these, then, among the intrusive images that went through her mind when she imagined John and his lover in bed?

"Yes, and then some. I imagine she did all the dirty things he wanted with a smile," she said sarcastically.

To help her sort through some complicated feelings, I wondered aloud if Frannie wasn't envious of this woman's imagined lack of inhibition. I asked her to consider whether John wanted to control her in bed to counter his inability to control her in life—to balance out their typical dynamic? And I proposed that penetrating him might feel so erotic to him that she might feel extremely potent. My comments struck home.

"I'd like to see John's face if I proposed that now," she said. "I'd blow his mind, I'm sure. I think my libido has always been based on what would happen to me. I've never actively thought about doing stuff to him. I controlled every mild sexual encounter with every boy before getting married because sex was something that could easily get out of control, I thought. Funny, isn't it—that it's out of control now? When John asked me about these weird—well, weird to me—ideas, I'm sure I shut him out further."

Desire can be fed by giving pleasure as well as receiving it. Stroking and caressing are like fanning the sparks of a fire. Everyone around gets warm once the flame becomes a roaring blaze. Until recently, Frannie had felt obligated to touch John. She had let her resentment of this "duty" interfere with really watching what she accomplished in him. As a young lover, she had been astounded by his penis and how it changed under her touch. But defensively, over the years, she had let her wonder and joy over her power cease as their multitude of relational hurts, big and small, had pulled them apart.

Sex after an affair can be the hottest sex of a person's life, according to some couples. Sometimes the affair gives both partners permission to blow the doors off their previously boxed-in sexuality. Long-repressed emotions come roiling forward in the aftermath of discovery, clearing away the dead undergrowth of withheld resentments. In rage, they often find courage to demand what they want sexually or act with abandon as a result of the jealousy they feel toward that third party and the experiences he or she had with their spouse. Seeing the potential demise of the relationship anyway, they return to the "why the hell not?" attitude of early lovers.

Frannie was jealous that John had experienced sex with other partners. Fortunately, she wasn't inclined to have a retaliatory affair, and I suggested that she use the opportunity of their "new" sexual relationship to try out things she might have been anxious about before or to experiment with her own fantasies.

She admitted that although she hadn't had fantasies for years, she did have them now. "But even that makes me angry," she said ruefully. "He had all this fabulous sex with her and now I change and he gets all this fabulous sex with me. It's unfair. It's like he wins and gets everything he wants and I just get hurt."

I risked challenging her hurt pride. "I'm not condoning what he did, but what would it have taken, Frannie, for the two of you to have started having fabulous sex at this age, then? Give me another scenario! And he hasn't had everything he wanted, not for years. And you told me yourself, he's changing emotionally too. Forget about him; what about you? Can you really live with that dull routine you described for the rest of your life just to get back at him?"

"I don't know." She exhaled with a pout. "He should have screamed and hollered and dragged me to a sex therapist instead of having an affair! For God's sake, that's where we are now."

Resolution of her ambivalent feelings took time and more couples work as well. Her rage and grief needed to be expressed before she could think about her own eroticism. A woman with less personal integrity might have hung on to her desire for revenge and cut off her nose to spite her face. In a later session, an impish look flashed over her face as she joked, "Shoot, I'm going to go home and tie him up and spank him, I think. I'll see how he likes it. He's been bad, bad, bad. While I'm at it, I'm going to call our last therapist and tell her off."

I laughed at the return of her sense of humor and hoped she'd do what she said. Then I encouraged her to call and tell the other therapist that her comment about breasts had really hurt Frannie and made her self-conscious. Knowing the professionalism of my colleague, I trusted that this would give Frannie some satisfaction.

Red, White, and Betrayed

Margarite called in urgent need of an appointment soon after Michael, her military husband, had returned from his deployment in Iraq. The pain in her voice was so palpable that I could guess what was going on.

She was a young brunette in a cotton shift dress and a thin sweater over her shoulders, and he was young too, dressed in khakis and a white T-shirt with his hair buzzed short. Their faces were solemn, and dark circles ringed her eyes. She looked tortured. With anguished intensity, she started the conversation by telling me that some girl had called Michael's cell phone, and that she had picked up.

"She wanted to know who I was. Who I am? I want to know who the hell she is!"

Michael sat silently, defiantly, on the couch. This was going to be a long session. To break the ice but not force him into a corner, I asked him how long he had been deployed.

"Eight months, ma'am," he answered with a southern twang, straightening on his cushion. Minimal information, I thought. I grimaced internally as I imagined him thinking, *Let the interrogation begin*. No ice broken.

Margarite couldn't contain herself any longer. "Last night was horrible. It was the worst night of my life. I think I flew at Michael at some point, because he just wouldn't tell me what was going on. I slapped him and tried to scratch him."

Finding out about a partner's affair can bring out the worst undisciplined behavior in even the most mature people. But physical violence always reflects severe deterioration of equilibrium, and nothing justifies it. Anxious to measure his temper, especially after the stresses of war, I asked her how he had responded. She said he'd caught her arms and held her off, then he'd taken the keys and left for a few hours. When he returned, she was in bed.

"I got up several times to try and get him to talk, but he wouldn't," she accused, shooting him a withering glance.

Nobody had gotten any sleep that night. Although I wanted to give Michael the benefit of the doubt, I suspected he'd had an affair and didn't have a clue as to how to break the news. It's usually therapeutic bad form to separate a couple right when an affair is discovered because there have already been too many secrets. But I knew that if I didn't connect with this young soldier, the work would be a lost cause. Since I had spoken with Margarite the day before, I hoped she might trust me to do what seemed best for a short while. I asked her if she could leave the room for fifteen minutes while I talked with Michael alone. Bitterly, she left the room with the door wide open.

After getting up to shut the door, I turned to Michael and said quietly, "So you get back from hell and now you're in it again," and I waited.

Several minutes of silence passed. Finally, leaning forward with elbows on his knees, he put his head in his hands. "I fucked up."

"Tell me," I said.

"There was this girl who was a civilian but worked at the base before I deployed. She wasn't, ah, how should I say this, a nice girl. Sexy as hell, though. I was anxious about going overseas, and one night about a week before I left, we had sex. She didn't mean anything to me, I swear. She emailed me a couple of times and I guess she figured out I was back. I really thought I'd never see her again."

It was an old story. I could picture a scared young cadet dumping his fright in some last fling with someone he didn't think he needed to respect, someone who would absorb his bad feelings; someone not Margarite, someone not his pristine, unsullied bride. It hadn't been right, but unfortunately, such situations are common. We ask our young service people to go into war and shut off their feelings and weaknesses long enough to get the job done. Marriages that need those very emotions to thrive are often casualties. It worried me that the pressure had led to him breaking his marital vows. It worried me that he could say the other girl didn't mean anything when her effort at contact suggested she felt otherwise. But this also pointed to the fact that the affair was probably more about him than about either woman as an individual.

After All I've Done for You

In the meantime, Margarite had done her duty too. She had been uprooted and transplanted more than once to support her husband's military career. These last eight months, she had bravely waited and prayed for Michael's return, every day afraid that he might not make it. She'd sent sexy emails and perfumed letters and her whole family had sent care packages. To be confronted with this infidelity after all her pining was a huge slap in the face.

"Margarite will never be able to handle this," he added. "She's fragile. It'll kill her."

His worry about her mental health showed his attachment to her, and at least it was a clue about why he had been silent the night before.

I brought Margarite back into the room and asked Michael to repeat what he'd told me. She cried for some time before the session was over.

When they returned for their second session a week later, Margarite was more wooden and quiet. The good news was that knowing about the affair hadn't killed her and that he was talking. Michael filled me in.

"It's been a rough few days. Margarite wanted to know all about it and wanted to know how the sex compared to ours. Now she's angry about what I've told her. She's also threatening to leave and go to her mother's."

In a flat, depressed voice, Margarite added, "I'm a dud in bed, he said."

Michael refuted her. "No, I did not say that. Sex has always been a point of contention for us, definitely. I want more of it and want it to be wilder, but that's not really the reason I slept with Teresa."

"Great, now she has a name," Margarite replied with sarcasm. "I thought she was just some bad girl who sucked all the nervous feelings out of you, not 'Teresa.'"

To me, she continued, "When I first heard her voice on the phone, I was frantic, but now I just feel hollow. You know, I'd heard all the stories of wives on base whose husbands had cheated, but I never thought I'd be one of them. I thought we were too in love. I guess I'm more the fool."

Margarite's biting comments and depression were understandable for someone whose sexual self-esteem and marital ideals had been devastated. Humiliation often overwhelms women who've just learned of an affair. They believe that they've been passed over for someone better, sexier, or more lovable.

"If I were stronger, I'd leave him, not just hate him."

Her lack of strength and autonomy made her feel as though she were trapped in the marriage. Her family would be disappointed if she left him, she said. She'd feel like a failure. God, and Uncle Sam needed her to love her man, come what may.

With no more than the superficial motivation of pleasing her parents and avoiding the stigma of separation, Margarite wasn't really staying in the marriage for herself. Nonetheless, she resumed sexual relations with Michael. At first, she cringed when he tried to touch her, but then she put on a show while making love, acting enthusiastic, pretending that she was really enjoying sex. She mistakenly believed that the only reason Michael had the affair was that he craved better sex—so that's what she tried to give him. Better sex was the only identifiable piece of the affair she could allow herself to understand. However, seeing his fear and weakness would have meant he wasn't her knight in shining armor. The more she performed, the less she felt, and her libido plummeted. Feeling good and being immersed in the moment would mean attaching to her husband emotionally again, and she couldn't trust that connection anymore.

I confronted her disastrous lack of decisiveness. She was still angry, I argued, so why try to merge before she felt trust again? Michael even confirmed that he was content to wait for sex until she was more ready. But her own dependency and insecurity led her to need this premature joining. What Michael had relayed about her fragility became more evident now, and I encouraged him to push for what he needed in terms of a whole and resilient partner. He balked at making any counterdemands, already feeling too guilt-ridden to ask for anything for himself. He and Margarite were mutually dependent; two halves trying to make up a whole. But without future growth as individuals, either of them in this young marriage might grab a third party in an attempt to stabilize matters when the going got rough. Therapy is a healthy way to bring in a neutral third party that also strengthens a marriage. Both Michael and Margarite needed to develop their own sense of purpose in the world not defined by the government or their parents. They needed lots of practice at communicating their real feelings and wishes. Unfortunately, they left treatment soon afterward. They were satisfied to have what was, in my opinion, a return to the status quo, and not genuine rehabilitation.

At any stage in a relationship, while our commitment to our partner should be permanent, we have to know that we can stand on our own two feet. We must have sufficient autonomy in order to have something to give. We must know our erotic self enough to have something to demand. The repression of libido is natural when an affair is first discovered and for some time thereafter. Healing sexually afterward requires a full decision to leave or to stay based on a renegotiation of the marriage that better suits both partners' needs. Wounds over the specific sexual rejection have to be assuaged through her partner's remorse. Sex itself must often be reconfigured. Barring the pathology of an involved partner's lack of conscience or sense of entitlement to having both spouse and mistress, the best result of this painful situation can be an opportunity for both parties to gain a more intimate understanding.

Help Yourself

1. What agreements do you and your partner have about feelings of attraction to someone else? Suggestion: Promise each other that if a serious attraction to another arises, you will tell either your partner, a friend who values your marriage, or a therapist.

2. If either partner has had an affair, what were the marital disappointments for each party prior to the crisis?

3. Describe your sexual life prior to the affair. What needed changing to make it fulfilling for both partners?

CHAPTER EIGHTEEN

When "No" Means "I Don't Love You Anymore"

When a marriage is dying, sex has often been absent, infrequent, or utilitarian for years. Perhaps this is what scares us when intimacy dries up: we worry that it means the marriage is in peril, the man is wrong for us, or maybe life isn't going to be as wonderful as we'd hoped. Fortunately, most of the time our marriage can be saved, the man is right for us even if he's not the shining knight we'd cracked him up to be, and life is both terrible and wonderful, with most of it falling somewhere between ordinary and quite good.

It's difficult to say when a marriage ends. The first fight we have stuns us from our bubble of happiness and idealization. Should we have known then that it wasn't right? But all spouses fight, all marriages have dark days, and all couples fantasize about how great it would be to have a really understanding partner. Marriage is difficult and a wise teacher once told me that most come to the breaking point at least once.

Often, one spouse uses the fuel of an affair to jettison out of the orbit of the marriage. Every once in a while someone looks hard and close at their relationship and painfully concludes that it's not enough, that there's not enough happiness to be wrung from it. Partners move forward in life in separate time frames. If children are involved, couples may stay together way past the time the relationship provided a healthy place for their kids to be nurtured. Economic considerations force many women to stay in soul- and libido-killing marriages. Blame is hurled. And for whatever the reason, leaving is always painful.

Sex is a private marker for how things are going in our heart of hearts. We've talked about how low libido is often caused by resentment. Sometimes we need to ask ourselves tough questions to figure out if our problems in the bedroom really are a sign that the relationship can't be fixed.

Leaving Is Tough

Certainly, when a hand has been raised in violence, it's hard to experience that same hand giving pleasure. Destructive anger, rage, and jealousy that intimidates a woman or her children is unacceptable. Addictions that wipe out the family resources of patience, energy, or money might only respond to separation. Repeated infidelities without repentance obviously strikes at the heart of sex. Decisions about these kinds of marriages can be difficult but are often more clear-cut. True, it seems couples leave each other over sexual incompatibilities, but the real reasons can be more complex. Low desire may be just a warning sign of the heart's fading commitment.

At twenty-nine, Tracy was starting to feel the dread of turning thirty. Depressed and worn down, she came into treatment wondering if her marriage to Frank was worth saving. She wanted children but confided that she wasn't sure about bringing them into this union.

Their relationship had started passionately with the best sex she had ever had. Frank's energy to please her in bed seemed endless. Many weekends were devoted to making love and lounging in bed. Sex was like a drug to Frank, calming him and helping him function. The first time Tracy turned him down, however, he had threatened to break up. It was the first time she saw through to his fragile psyche, and at the time she felt love and sympathy.

Little things she had ignored when they were dating, however, grew into larger patterns of selfishness and bullying. Once, after their engagement, when he had come to her parents' house for dinner, he had gotten drunk and criticized her mother's cooking. Her father had sternly told her to think twice before she married him, but in an effort to remain independent, she had dismissed his advice as judgmental. Later Frank accused her of wanting an old boyfriend after they had run into him at a wedding. But they repaired their argument with hot makeup sex that evening. When Tracy moved into his apartment right before the wedding, Frank hadn't helped with the lifting, transporting, cleaning, or unpacking. In fact, he seemed irritated that she had brought so much stuff. At the time she felt that she might be expecting too much and rationalized that everyone had flaws.

The first years of marriage were increasingly difficult. Frank started to call her cell phone at all hours of the day demanding to know what she was doing and whom she was with. He would not share his financial information and said she was snooping when she asked about specific credit-card bills that appeared, alarmingly, in both their names. Paranoia governed their mutual state of mind.

Sexually, he had suggested they tell each other their fantasies. When Tracy did this, he held it against her, and shockingly—she thought he was kidding at first—called her a whore. When he got really angry, she started to feel afraid even though he'd never hit her. If she was enthusiastic in her responses, he would wonder aloud if she was thinking of someone else. If she had trouble or couldn't climax, he would often leave the bed disgusted with her performance and claim she must not love him. He would taunt that she had given her best sex to other men and pout that he'd been left with a used-up woman. Their intimate life seemed to crystalize the bind she felt in the marriage as a whole. He didn't really want to be with her and he couldn't let her out of his sight.

After a few years of this, Tracy wished she could never have sex with him again even though she wouldn't dare say no. His controlling behavior and criticism smothered her desire. His anger made every day tense.

"I don't understand why he is angry all the time," she began. "I'm the last person on the planet who would cheat on him; I never even want sex. In fact, I wish sex wasn't invented at this point. I'm tired of fighting about it. The men he's jealous of meant very little to me. In fact, I really didn't have that much sex before I met Frank."

Tracy had parents who cared about her. She'd had a stable upbringing. Divorce was not part of her family's heritage and she took her commitment seriously. Frank's father had died early and his mother was forced to search for work. She'd left him in the care of his grandparents, who did not want the responsibility of a toddler. He grew up neglected and fell in with a rough crowd. His pervasive anger was the residue of his disturbed childhood attachments and rejections. Sex triggered all his longing for holding and loving but also his fears of being dependent again. He projected those fears onto Tracy, which left her feeling helpless, needy, and bad most of the time.

I was concerned for Tracy's safety if Frank were to become abusive so we developed a plan for her to leave the home if his anger started to escalate. Frank's trauma of abandonment and loss was mostly unconscious to him; he remembered what happened but couldn't see how this changed anything in the present. He had come to a session or two but was only interested in Tracy becoming a more perfect sexual partner, not in how his history was driving her away.

Eventually Tracy decided that she was working on a problem that was too big for her to solve. Her own failings in the marriage contributed to her guilty feelings about leaving and she felt embarrassed at admitting to her parents how difficult her marital problems had become. Low libido signaled her own rage at being the repository for her husband's bad feelings and cruelty. I saw it as a healthy response, protecting her from Frank's impossible sexual demands and emotional mess. Though she did not want to be one more person in his life who abandoned him, Tracy now knew the future she wanted wasn't possible with Frank. Eventually, with the help of her father, she left.

Growing Apart

At sixty and nearing retirement, Sidney, an African-American, was a popular dance instructor at our local state college. Her gray hair was cropped, and she wore exotic eye makeup and bold jewelry. Her still-lithe limbs were evident through close-fitting, thin layers of cotton and cashmere. She and her husband, Nathan, Caucasian and a pilot, had traveled the world in their youth collecting art and visiting theaters. Married in the early 1970s, Sidney had warned Nathan—then in his campus activist days before he entered the air force—that their marriage had to be based on the two of them, not a zealous fantasy about how the world ought to live. America had been hard on the young couple, but they had lived in the West, where there seemed to be more tolerance for their interracial union, until Sidney's aging mother had needed her to come home to the South.

Grieving the loss of her mother and her newly empty nest, Sidney relayed that over the years her and Nathan's ideals had become jaded and their bodies less passionate. They had tried couples therapy several times, but Nathan seemed to find fault with each therapist whenever his contributions to the problems were pointed out. With the children gone, much of the day-to-day stressors were also gone. Sidney's marriage had died and she had come to therapy for its epitaph.

Sex was problematic, she began, hoping that I might be able to save their relationship if only I could salvage their intimate life. I asked her if there had ever been a time of greater sexual connection.

"Oh, sure," Sidney replied. "In college, sex was fast and furious.

We got together in a town and time when it wasn't quite as acceptable to shack up. And our interracial relationship was still fairly taboo, so I suppose sex had a racy edge. He loved my body and how flexible I was. He'd gush over my skin. Basically, I wasn't his mother and he was trying to get as far away from her as he could. My warm black skin was a clear contrast to her ice-cold rejection. His worship of my body made me fall in love with him.

"Then he went to Vietnam and came back an absolutely hollow soul. I could barely recognize him. He had nightmares and flashbacks before returning vets were ever diagnosed with post-traumatic stress syndrome. I know now that's what it was. I guess the evil and pain he saw overwhelmed him and he needed something concrete to hang on to—but it was no longer me. When he left, he wanted to change the world. He returned wanting to make money.

"At first, I thought it might be fun to travel with him, and to some extent it was. But I really wanted him back—I wanted my romantic, fanatical idealist back.

"I've tried talking to Nathan and asking him what he wants from our marriage and our life," she ended.

"What did he say?" I asked.

"Basically nothing. It's a little like trying to have a conversation with an angry teenager. You get a grunt, a shrug, or completely ignored. He just looks at me and walks away."

Then what? "I've yelled, I've written letters, I've pleaded. I think I've given up now. How do you work on things if your partner just won't respond?"

She continued: "Really, shortly after our wedding, things changed sexually. I'd complain about how it was all so different than what we'd had and he would pout in silence. Nothing I said could reach him. He heard my pining as criticism of his performance—a mortal wound. Then, when I couldn't come at all, he would complain about it in a really critical way—sort of to get me back. I wasn't like the girls before me. I wasn't wet when he touched me. But God, he only touched me right when he wanted sex and I was supposed to turn on instantly. I'd tell him I needed more time, but he'd never get it. More time meant an extra minute or two. It's been over a decade since I've had an orgasm with him and now I don't want one with him. I turn him away because he turns me away."

Trying to figure out his perspective without him there, I asked what his criticisms of her were. "Not enough sex certainly is top of the list. He also thinks I spend too much money, but we have the money. Our retirement is secure and his parents will probably leave him more money than he'll know what to do with, and they're in their late eighties now."

Sidney went on: "What really gets me is how after days and days of silence, he can just reach over and grope me in the dark and actually expect sex!"

"What do you do when he reaches for you?" I wondered aloud.

Sidney exclaimed, "I've yelled, I've ignored, I've said no, I've said yes, I've bargained with him . . . you get the picture. No matter what I do, nothing changes! It's not that I don't have any sexual feelings—unfortunately, I do—but I can't muster any feelings for Nathan. And the sex is always the same. If I didn't know any better, I'd say his head is a block of wood. Nothing gets through to him. He doesn't see sex as my gift of love to him. He only notices when I say no and sees my rejection as withholding. He doesn't think that his silence and lack of affection is anywhere near as bad as my not wanting to have sex. But God, I just can't stand it some days—I feel worse after having sex. And I feel sick at heart because I can imagine a relationship that is warm at our stage of life. I can imagine being with a man whose touch is gentle, curious, and exciting. I imagine a man who wants to know me at this age—my mind and my body! Imagination is really a terrible thing. Please don't tell me I just need to do something spontaneous or new."

Sidney's frustration was poignant. A passionate love affair turned cold because of the wounds of a war beyond their control and the wounds from his rejecting mother still unexamined. She knew that sex could still be good and a relationship be loving, but she couldn't turn the tide in her existing marriage. Nathan's withdrawal into an empty shell translated to "I can't, don't, and won't share my feelings."

When he had become a commercial pilot, she had oohed and aahed over the treasures he brought home from his flights. They had traveled to Tahiti on a whim. "But you know, once you have children, that kind of freedom doesn't really happen," Sidney continued. "Then, in my loneliness, I wanted real involvement with my classes, my students, and our community. He didn't get it. He'd given up on the world. And he became this spoiled baby who wanted all my attention and begrudged what I gave to our daughters. His judgment and withdrawal brought a gloom that hung over the house when he was home between trips. We were happier without him. We fought over so many issues I've lost count. Sometimes he'd be directly critical, like about sex. My attempts to make him happy were often misconstrued as manipulation. I couldn't win for losing. And I've tried. I've blamed the war, the government, prejudice, and his stony mother, but I've not been able to find a way through to him."

Couples therapy had failed. He'd rejected her theories of PTSD and ignored her when she begged for him to think about medication for his depression. She'd asked for what she needed emotionally and sexually; she was exhausted from her efforts. After I heard all of this, it was clear to me—and clearer to Sidney.

"Your marriage is over," I reflected calmly.

There Must Be More

In response, Sidney said, "Yes. And I'm sixty. I don't have forever in front of me. Maybe I thought I was too old and I should just live the 'good life' with this man and count my blessings. But I can't imagine going through the rest of my life with so little connection. The girls will be devastated, I think, but they have their own full lives and we see precious little of them now. Does all this make me selfish? Probably."

It sounded like psychic survival to me. I asked if there was someone else. Often when a person has come to this point, they've already formed an alliance elsewhere.

"No, there isn't. But I'm not dead. I see interesting men around. Dancing has kept me in shape and I have a grandmother who's near a hundred and still a spitfire. I meet men at work and at church who have been divorced or widowed and they seem to have a part inside that is still alive. Perhaps they'll ask a question or two about me or my life and I think, 'Huh, that's more interest than my husband has shown in a year.' There isn't anyone special.

I wouldn't even let my fantasies go in that direction. I'm a Methodist and we do things in order. The first order of business is to let go of the marriage. Next order is to enjoy being just me for a while and maybe then enjoy the process of dating again."

It's hard to know whether long-standing sexual problems (entangled in relational problems) can be solved or are indications of a closed heart. No one wants to give up on a marriage that they have invested with hope and time. Sidney's low libido was relationship-specific. Her husband was not interested in her or in life in general. Nathan's resolute silence at this stage had left the marriage cold. She knew before she came to treatment what she wanted but apparently needed to say it out loud and hear someone else say it out loud. For Tracy, on the other hand, low sexual desire came from living with a man who was threatened by the very thing he wanted. At some point, though, whether for psychic survival, relief, or the chance at considerably more happiness, an individual may have to evaluate whether to continue working on the problem or whether to let the relationship go.

Help Yourself

1. Identify your part in your behaviors and withheld behaviors that contribute to your marital problems.

2. Describe the patterns of intimacy reflected by your parents or caretakers in your childhood and how they impacted you.

3. What models of connection, sexually and relationally, was your spouse shown in his childhood?

4. What unresolved traumas, infidelities, or conflicts are between you and your partner?

5. Seek a marital therapist to discuss the viability of recovery from your existing difficulties.

Sexual desire is the fruit and fuel for a happy marriage. It is the ordinary holiday that sets moments apart from the monotony of life. At the same time we feed our partner, we are nourished in a deeply intimate way. Allowing ourselves the vulnerable need for touch, affection, pleasure, and excitement satisfies our primitive and adult needs for attachment in a way that nothing else can.

As we've seen, a woman needs the reliability of orgasm, good technique, and some skillful seduction to feel motivated to have sex. She must ask for and teach her partner how to touch her in favorite and practical ways. She must know what makes her feel good. Believing her husband's commitment to please her means she continues to tell him what feels good, even if he forgets once in a while in a passionate moment. Courageously, she must fight for her different arousal pattern. She must trust the relationship and her own body to submit to lovemaking without worrying that she is "taking too long."

Relational problems have to be resolved for a woman to stay alive sexually. Emotional pursuers and sexual distancers can grow in their capacity to connect without having to wait for their partner to change. We can dramatically change the relationship simply by changing our part in the problem. Because we love, we must also learn to give even when it makes us afraid that our needs will be overlooked. Because we respect ourselves, we require fairness and we make clear requests. We risk "going first," to offer love. Our partner needs and feels our love for some time before they feel ready to make changes. Balancing our needs with our partner's needs, we form a special relationship between us that takes priority over all others. Sometimes we must recognize pervasive patterns of cruelty or sadism and end the relationship.

We can learn to see sex as a way to connect and feel good. Sometimes we can choose to be close physically as a prelude to emotional closeness, instead of the other way around, and let physical stimulation turn on our desire.

We take ownership of ourselves when we initiate sex. We pick up sexual clues from our daily interactions and use our own fantasies to build sexual feelings that we bring to bed. Risking novelty and variety brings just the right sort of anxiety that makes sex exciting. Prioritizing sex, pleasure, and relaxation in our marriage over the endless demands of life ensures that our relationship is both stable and exciting. Contrary to the media illusion, all good, enduring sexual relationships require a great deal of work. We must bring time, energy, analysis, and creativity to the sexual relationship in order to continue to feel desire.

We can heal the relational blueprint we've inherited from

childhood that gives us the wrong ideas about sex and committed intimacy. We can be free from repeating those unresolved hurts by becoming conscious of what they were, and how they limited our sexual freedom and relational happiness. With a fresh look at our relationship, we can choose to risk trying different and more exciting ways to live and escape the depression, addictions, and hopelessness of poor histories.

We can leave a new legacy for our daughters by teaching them that sexual passion is an essential component of life. Telling them that sex feels great helps them accept their sexual feelings as good. We can teach them about safe sex—for the body and the heart. We can listen to their intensity about their first love with seriousness and careful reflection.

We must commit to our sexual health with regular gynecological appointments, attend to problems of discomfort promptly, research our options for menopause, and rigorously seek medical expertise for help.

When we're sexually alive, it infuses the rest of our life with joy.

· NOTES ·

Chapter One

1. Rosemary Basson, "A Model of Women's Sexual Arousal," *Journal of Sex & Marital Therapy* 28 (2002): 1–10; doi: 10.1080/009262302317250963.
2. Scharff modeled the phrase "good-enough sex" on D. W. Winnicott's phrase "good-enough mothering." David Scharff, *The Sexual Relationship* (Northvale, NJ: Jason Aronson, Inc., 1998), 132.

Chapter Three

1. Daniel Bergner, "What Do Women Want?," *New York Times*, January 22, 2009.
2. Carol Gilligan, *In a Different Voice: Psychological Theory and Women's Development* (Cambridge, MA: Harvard University Press, 1993), 21. The full quote is "Thus while Kohlberg's subject worries about people interfering with each other's rights, this woman worries about 'the possibility of omission, of your not helping others when you could help them.'"
3. Carol Gilligan, *The Birth of Pleasure: A New Map of Love* (New York: Vintage Books, 2002), Kindle edition.

Chapter Five

1. Caitlin Flanagan, *To Hell with All That: Loving and Loathing Our Inner Housewife* (New York: Little, Brown, 2006), 30.

Chapter Six

1. Daniel Bergner, "What Do Women Want?," *New York Times*, January 22, 2009.

Chapter Eight

1. David Scharff, *The Sexual Relationship* (Northvale, NJ: Jason Aronson, Inc., 1998), 109–126.

2. Rosemary Basson, "A Model of Women's Sexual Arousal," *Journal of Sex & Marital Therapy* 28 (2002): 1–10; doi: 10.1080/009262302317250963.

3. Carol Gilligan, *In a Different Voice: Psychological Theory and Women's Development* (Cambridge, MA: Harvard University Press, 1993), 163.

4. Scharff, 127–190.

5. Deborah Tolman, *Dilemmas of Desire: Teenage Girls Talk About Sexuality* (Cambridge, MA: Harvard University Press, 2002), 176.

6. Mary Pipher, *Reviving Ophelia* (New York: Penguin Books, 1994), chapter fourteen. Tolman, 175.

7. Tolman, 111.

8. Scharff, 101.

Chapter Nine

1. David Scharff, *The Sexual Relationship* (Northvale, NJ: Jason Aronson, Inc., 1998), 7.

Chapter Ten

1. Bahroo, B. "Special Issue: Child Protection in the 21st Century: Pedophilia: Psychiatric Insights." Family Court Review 41, 4 (October 2003) 497-507.

2. Jody Davies and Mary Frawley, *Treating the Adult Survivor of Childhood Sexual Abuse* (New York: Basic Books, 1994), 67.

3. "National Child Abuse Statistics," *Childhelp*, accessed July 1, 2012, http://www.childhelp.org/pages/statistics.

4. Wendy Maltz, *The Sexual Healing Journey: A Guide for Survivors of Sexual Abuse* (New York: HarperCollins, 1991), 251.

5. Davies and Frawley, 67.

Chapter Eleven

1. Richard Balon, "SSRI-Associated Sexual Dysfunction," *American Journal of Psychiatry* 163 (2006):1504–1509; doi:10.1176/appi.ajp.163.9.1504.

Chapter Thirteen

1. "Androgens, Antidepressants, and Other Drugs on Which the Jury's Still Out," *North American Menopause Society*, accessed April 1, 2006, http://www.menopause.org/SHM/5otherdrugs.aspx.

2. Dona Caine-Francis, *Managing Menopause Beautifully: Physically, Emotionally, and Sexually.* Westport, CT: Praeger Publishers, 2008, 2.

3. Clarisa R. Gracia, et al., "Hormones and Sexuality During Transition to Menopause," *Obstetrics & Gynecology* 109:4 (2007): 831-840.

4. *Hot Flash Havoc*, DVD, directed by Marc Bennett (United States: Hot Flash Havoc, 2010).

5. "Testosterone Reference Ranges in Adults," *Quest Diagnostics*, December 2011; http://www.questdiagnostics.com/hcp/intguide/EndoMetab/Gen_Misc/ Testosterone/Table%201.pdf.

6. Topiwala, Shehzad. "Testosterone." Medline Plus, 2012, www.nlm.nih.gov/ medlineplus/ency/article/003707.htm (August 28, 2012).

7. Glenn D. Braunstein, "Commentary: The Endocrine Society Clinical Practice Guideline and the North American Menopause Society Position Statement on Androgen Therapy in Women: Another One of Yogi's Forks," *Journal of Clinical Endocrinology & Metabolism* 92:11 (2007): 4091–4093. Jan L. Shifren, et al., "Transdermal Testosterone Treatment in Women with Impaired Sexual Function After Oophorectomy," *New England Journal of Medicine* 343 (2000): 682–688.

8. Jan L. Shifren and Isaac Schiff, "Role of Hormone Therapy in the Management of Menopause," *Obstetrics & Gynecology* 115 (2010): 839–855.

9. Caine-Francis, 54.

10. Christiane Northrup, *The Wisdom of Menopause: Creating Physical and Emotional Health and Healing During the Change* (New York: Bantam, 2006), 170.

11. Shifren and Schiff, 847.

12. *Hot Flash Havoc.*

13. Kent Holtorf, "The Bioidentical Hormone Debate: Are Bioidentical Hormones (Estradiol, Estriol, and Progesterone) Safer or More Efficacious than Commonly Used Synthetic Versions in Hormone Replacement Therapy?" *Postgraduate Medicine* 121:1 (2009): 1–13.

14. Esther Perel, *Mating in Captivity* (New York: HarperCollins Publishers Inc., 2006), 170.

15. Daniel Bergner, "What Do Women Want?," *New York Times*, January 22, 2009.

16. Christiane Northrup, *The Secret Pleasures of Menopause* (Carlsbad, CA: Hay House, 2008), 7.

17. John E. Buster, et al., "Testosterone Patch for Low Sexual Desire in Surgically Menopausal Women: A Randomized Trial" *Obstetrics & Gynecology* 105:5 (2006): 944–952; doi:10.1097/01.AOG.0000158103.27672.0d.

Chapter Fourteen

1. Andrew Goldstein, Caroline Pukall, and Irwin Goldstein, *When Sex Hurts: A Woman's Guide to Banishing Sexual Pain* (New York: Da Capo Lifelong Books, 2011), 152.

2. Ibid., 157.

3. Ibid., 105–107.

4. Andrew T. Goldstein and Lara Burrows, "Vulvodynia." *Journal of Sexual Medicine* 5 (2008): 5–15; doi:10.1111/j.1743-6109.2007.00679.x.

5. S. Wills et al., "Effects of Vaginal Estrogens on Serum Estradiol Levels in Post-menopausal Breast Cancer Survivors Taking an Aromatase Inhibitor or a Selective Estrogen Receptor Modulator," *Cancer Research* 69 (2009): 806; doi: 10.1158/0008-5472.SABCS-09-806.

6. J. E. Dew, B. G. Wren, and J. A. Eden, "Tamoxifen, Hormone Receptors and Hormone Replacement Therapy in Women Previously Treated for Breast Cancer: a Cohort Study," *Climacteric* 5 (2002): 151–155.

7. Ellen Bernard and Myrtle Wilhite, "Adult Toys," *A Woman's Touch*; http://www.a-womans-touch.com/.

Chapter Fifteen

1. David Scharff, *The Sexual Relationship* (Northvale, NJ: Jason Aronson, Inc., 1998), 133.

2. Harville Hendrix and Helen Hunt, *Receiving Love: Transform Your Relationship by Letting Yourself Be Loved* (New York, NY: Atria Books, 2004), 35.

Chapter Seventeen

1. David Scharff, *The Sexual Relationship* (Northvale, NJ: Jason Aronson, Inc., 1998), 202.

· BIBLIOGRAPHY ·

"Androgens, Antidepressants, and Other Drugs on Which the Jury's Still Out."
  North American Menopause Society. Accessed April 1, 2006. http://www.menopause
  .org/SHM/5otherdrugs.aspx.
Basson, Rosemary. "A Model of Women's Sexual Arousal." *Journal of Sex & Marital
  Therapy* 28 (2002): 1–10. doi: 10.1080/009262302317250963.
Balon, Richard. "SSRI-Associated Sexual Dysfunction." *American Journal of Psychiatry*
  163 (2006): 1504–1509. doi:10.1176/appi.ajp.163.9.1504.
Barbach, Lonnie. *The Erotic Edge: 22 Erotic Stories for Couples.* New York: Plume, 1994.
Belenky, Mary; Clinchy, Blythe; and Nancy Goldberger. *Women's Ways of Knowing: The
  Development of Self, Voice, and Mind.* New York: Basic Books, 1986.
Bergner, Daniel. "What Do Women Want?" *New York Times,* January 22, 2009. www
  .nytimes.com.
Bernard, Ellen, and Myrtle Wilhite. "Adult Toys." *A Woman's Touch.* http://www
  .a-womans-touch.com/.
Betchen, Stephen J. *Intrusive Partners, Elusive Mates: The Pursuer-Distancer Dynamic in Cou-
  ples.* New York: Routledge, 2005.
Block, Joel D. *Secrets of Better Sex: A Noted Sex Therapist Reveals His Secrets to Passionate Sexual
  Fulfillment.* Paramus, NJ: Reward Books, 1996.
Braunstein, Glenn D. "Commentary: The Endocrine Society Clinical Practice
  Guideline and the North American Menopause Society Position Statement on
  Androgen Therapy in Women: Another One of Yogi's Forks." *Journal of Clinical
  Endocrinology & Metabolism* 92:11 (2007): 4091–4093.
Bright, Susie. *Full Exposure: Opening Up to Sexual Creativity and Erotic Expression.* San Fran-
  cisco: HarperSanFrancisco, 1999.
Buber, Martin. *I And Thou,* trans. Walter Kaufmann. New York: Touchstone, 1971.
Buster, John E.; Kingsberg, Sheryl A.; Aguirre, Oscar; Brown, Candace; Breaux,

Jeffrey G.; Buch, Akshay; Rodenberg, Cynthia A.; Wekselman, Kathryn; and Peter Casson. "Testosterone Patch for Low Sexual Desire in Surgically Menopausal Women: A Randomized Trial." *Obstetrics & Gynecology* 105:5 (2006): 944–952. doi:10.1097/01.AOG.0000158103.27672.0d.

Caine-Francis, Dona. *Managing Menopause Beautifully: Physically, Emotionally, and Sexually.* Westport, CT: Praeger Publishers, 2008.

Chalker, Rebecca. *The Clitoral Truth: The Secret World at Your Fingertips.* New York: Seven Stories Press, 2000.

Chivers, Meredith; Rieger, Gerulf; Latty, Elizabeth; and J. Michael Bailey. "A Sex Difference in the Specificity of Sexual Arousal." *Psychological Science* 15 (2004): 736–744. doi:10.1111/j.0956-7976.2004.00750.x.

Clulow, Christopher, ed. *Sex, Attachment and Couple Psychotherapy.* London: Karmac Books Ltd., 2009.

Davies, Jody M., and Mary G. Frawley. *Treating the Adult Survivor of Childhood Sexual Abuse.* New York: Basic Books, 1994.

Dew, J. E.; Wren, B. G.; and J. A. Eden. "Tamoxifen, Hormone Receptors and Hormone Replacement Therapy in Women Previously Treated for Breast Cancer: a Cohort Study." *Climacteric* 5 (2002): 151–155.

Firestone, Robert W.; Firestone, Lisa A.; and Joyce Catlett. *Sex and Love in Intimate Relationships.* Washington, D.C.: American Psychological Association, 2006.

Fisher, Helen. *Why We Love: The Nature and Chemistry of Romantic Love.* New York: Henry Holt and Company, 2004.

———. *Anatomy of Love: A Natural History of Mating, Marriage, and Why We Stray.* New York: Fawcett Books, 1992.

Flanagan, Caitlin. *To Hell with All That: Loving and Loathing Our Inner Housewife.* New York: Little, Brown and Company, 2006.

Forward, Susan. *Innocence and Betrayal: Overcoming the Legacy of Sexual Abuse.* 1992. Dove Entertainment Inc. Audiocassette.

Gabriel, Bonnie. *The Fine Art of Erotic Talk: How to Entice, Excite, and Enchant Your Lover With Words.* New York: Bantam Books, 1996.

Gilligan, Carol. *The Birth of Pleasure: A New Map of Love.* New York: Vintage Books, 2002.

———. *In A Different Voice: Psychological Theory and Women's Development.* Cambridge, MA: Harvard University Press, 1993.

Goldstein, Andrew, and Laura Burrows. "Vulvodynia." *Journal of Sexual Medicine* 5 (2008): 5–15. doi:10.1111/j.1743-6109.2007.00679.x.

Goldstein, Andrew; Pukall, Caroline; and Irwin Goldstein. *When Sex Hurts: A Woman's Guide to Banishing Sexual Pain.* New York: Da Capo Press, 2011.

Gottman, John M., and Nan Silver. *The Seven Principles for Making Marriage Work: A*

Practical Guide from the Country's Foremost Relationship Expert. New York: Three Rivers Press, 1999.

Gracia, Clarisa R.; Freeman, Ellen W.; Sammel, Mary D.; Lin, Hui; and Marjori Mogul. "Hormones and Sexuality During Transition to Menopause." *Obstetrics & Gynecology* 109:4 (2007): 831–840.

Hall, Kathryn. *Reclaiming Your Sexual Self: How You Can Bring Desire Back into Your Life.* Hoboken, NJ: John Wiley & Sons, 2004.

Hendrix, Harville, and Helen Hunt. *Receiving Love: Transform Your Relationship by Letting Yourself Be Loved.* New York: Atria Books, 2004.

Holtorf, Kent. "The Bioidentical Hormone Debate: Are Bioidentical Hormones (Estradiol, Estriol, and Progesterone) Safer or More Efficacious Than Commonly Used Synthetic Versions in Hormone Replacement Therapy?" *Postgraduate Medicine* 121:1 (2009): 1–13.

Hot Flash Havoc. DVD. Directed by Marc Bennett. 2010; United States: Hot Flash Havoc, 2010.

Huddleston, Mary, ed. *Celibate Loving: Encounter in Three Dimensions.* Ramsey, NJ: Paulist Press.

Hunter, Marianne. *Sex: A Book of Quotations.* New York: Barnes & Noble Books, 2003.

Johnson, Robert A. *She: Understanding Feminine Psychology.* New York: HarperPerennial, 1989.

————. *Owning Your Own Shadow: Understanding the Dark Side of the Psyche.* San Francisco: HarperSanFrancisco, 1991.

————. *We: Understanding the Psychology of Romantic Love.* New York: HarperCollins Publishers, 1983.

Johnson, Sue. *Hold Me Tight: Seven Conversations for a Lifetime of Love.* New York: Little, Brown and Company, 2008.

Kaplan, Helen S. *The Sexual Desire Disorders: Dysfunctional Regulation of Sexual Motivation.* Bristol, PA: Brunner/Mazel, 1995.

Karen, Robert. *Becoming Attached: First Relationships and How They Shape Our Capacity to Love.* New York: Oxford University Press, 1994.

Kaschak, Ellyn, and Leonore Tiefer, eds. *A New View of Women's Sexual Problems.* New York: Haworth Press, 2001.

Keesling, Barbara. *The Good Girl's Guide to Bad Girl Sex: An Indispensible Guide to Pleasure and Seduction.* New York: M. Evans and Company, 2001.

Kessler, David A. *The End of Overeating: Taking Control of the Insatiable American Appetite.* New York: Rodale, 2009.

Krychman, Michael L.; Kellogg, Susan; and Sandra Finestone. *100 Questions & Answers: About Breast Cancer Sensuality, Sexuality, and Intimacy.* Sudbury, MA: Jones & Bartlett Learning, 2011.

Lachkar, Joan. *The Narcissistic/Borderline Couple: A Psychoanalytic Perspective on Marital Treatment*. Bristol, PA: Brunner/Mazel, 1992.

Lamb, Sharon. *The Secret Lives of Girls: What Good Girls Really Do—Sex, Play, Aggression, and Their Guilt*. New York: Free Press, 2001.

Leiblum, Sandra R., and Raymond C. Rosen, eds. *Principles and Practice of Sexy Therapy: Update for the 1990s*. New York: Guilford Press, 1989.

Leiblum, Sandra R., and Judith Sachs. *Getting the Sex You Want: A Woman's Guide to Becoming Proud, Passionate and Pleased in Bed*. New York: ASJA Press, 2002.

Leiblum, Sandra R., ed. *Treating Sexual Desire Disorders: A Clinical Casebook*. New York: Guilford Press, 2010.

Love, Patricia, and Jo Robinson. *Hot Monogamy: Essential Steps to More Passionate, Intimate Lovemaking*. New York: Plume, 1994.

Love, Patricia. *How to Improve Your Marriage Without Talking About It*. New York: Three Rivers Press, 2008.

Maisano, Gina M. *Intimacy After Breast Cancer: Dealing With Your Body, Relationships and Sex*. Garden City Park, NY: Square One Publishers, 2010.

Maltz, Wendy. *The Sexual Healing Journey: A Guide for Survivors of Sexual Abuse*. New York: HarperCollins Publishers, 1991.

Masters, William H.; Johnson, Virginia E.; and Robert Kolodny. *On Sex and Human Loving*. Boston: Little, Brown & Company, 1982.

McCarthy, Barry W., and Emily J. McCarthy. *Rekindling Desire: A Step-by-Step Program to Help Low-Sex and No-Sex Marriages*. New York: Taylor & Francis Books, 2003.

Miller, J. B.; Jorden, J.; Stiver, I.; and Janet Surrey. *Women's Growth In Connection; Writings from the Stone Center*. New York: Guilford Press, 1991.

Mintz, Laurie B. *A Tired Woman's Guide to Passionate Sex: Reclaim Your Desire and Reignite Your Relationship*. Avon, MA: Adams Media, 2009.

Mitchell, Stephen A. *Can Love Last?: The Fate of Romance over Time*. New York: W. W. Norton & Company, 2002.

Morin, Jack. *The Erotic Mind: Unlocking the Inner Sources of Sexual Passion and Fulfillment*. New York: HarperCollins Publishers, 1995.

Northrup, Christiane. *The Wisdom of Menopause*. New York: Bantam Dell, 2001.

———. *The Secret Pleasures of Menopause*. Carlsbad, CA: Hay House, 2008.

Ogden, Gina. *The Return of Desire: A Guide to Rediscovering Your Sexual Passion*. Boston: Trumpeter Books, 2008.

Penner, Clifford, and Joyce Penner. *The Gift of Sex: A Guide to Sexual Fulfillment*. Nashville: W Publishing Group, 2003.

Perel, Esther. *Mating In Captivity: Reconciling the Erotic and the Domestic*. New York: HarperCollins Publishers, 2006.

Perry, Susan K. *Loving in Flow: How the Happiest Couples Get and Stay That Way*. Naperville, IL: Sourcebooks Casablanca, 2003.

Pipher, Mary. *Reviving Ophelia: Saving the Selves of Adolescent Girls.* New York: Penguin Books, 1994.

Pope, Kenneth S.; Sonne, Janet L.; and Jean Holroyd. *Sexual Feelings in Psychotherapy: Explorations for Therapists and Therapists-in-Training.* Washington, D.C.: American Psychological Association, 1993.

Reichman, Judith. *I'm Not in the Mood: What Every Woman Should Know About Improving Her Libido.* New York: Quill/William Morrow, 1998.

Rinehart, Paula. *Sex and the Soul of a Woman: How God Restores the Beauty of Relationship from the Pain of Regret.* Grand Rapids, MI: Zondervan, 2004.

Roach, Mary. *Boink: The Curious Coupling of Science and Sex.* New York: W. W. Norton & Company, 2008.

Rose, Tracy. "Weightism: How to Deal with Unfair Prejudice Against Obese People." April 2007. http://tracy-rose.suite101.com/weightism-a17783.

Rosenau, Douglas E. *A Celebration of Sex: A Guide to Enjoying God's Gift of Sexual Intimacy.* Nashville: Thomas Nelson, 2002.

Rosenau, Douglas E., Neel, Deborah C., and Ellen Fox. *A Celebration of Sex: Guidebook.* Maitland, FL: Xulon Press, 2007.

Sack, David A. *No More Secrets, No More Shame: Understanding Sexual Abuse and Emotional Disorders.* Washington, D.C.: PIA Press, 1990.

Sanford, John A. *The Invisible Partners: How the Male and Female in Each of Us Affects Our Relationships.* Mahwah, NJ: Paulist Press, 1980.

Scharff, David E. *The Sexual Relationship.* Northvale, NJ: Jason Aronson, 1982.

———. *Object Relations Couple Therapy.* Northvale, NJ: Jason Aronson, 1977.

Schnarch, David. *Passionate Marriage.* New York: Henry Holt and Company, 1997.

———. *Resurrecting Sex.* New York: HarperCollins Publishers, 2002.

Sewell, Joan. *I'd Rather Eat Chocolate: Learning to Love My Low Libido.* New York: Broadway Books, 2007.

"Sexual Health & Menopause: Changes in Hormone Levels." *North American Menopause Society.* June 13, 2011. http://www.menopause.org/SHM/2hormonelevels.aspx.

Sharpe, Shelia A. *The Ways We Love: A Developmental Approach to Treating Couples.* New York: Guilford Press, 2000.

Shifren, Jan L.; Braunstein, Glenn D.; Simon, James A.; Casson, Peter R.; Buster, John E.; Redmond, Geoffrey P.; Burki, Regula E.; Ginsburg, Elizabeth S.; Rosen, Raymond C.; Leiblum, Sandra R.; Caramelli, Kim E.; Jones, Kirtley P.; Daugherty, Claire A.; and Norman A. Mazer. "Transdermal Testosterone Treatment in Women with Impaired Sexual Function After Oophorectomy." *New England Journal of Medicine* 343 (2000): 682–688.

Shifren, Jan L., and Isaac Schiff. "Role of Hormone Therapy in the Management of Menopause." *Obstetrics & Gynecology* 115 (2010): 839–855.

Solot, Dorian, and Marshall Miller. *I Love Female Orgasm: An Extraordinary Orgasm Guide.* New York: Da Capo Press, 2007.

Steinberg, David, ed. *The Erotic Impulse: Honoring the Sensual Self.* New York: G. P. Putnam Sons, 1992.

Steiner, Claude M. *When a Man Loves a Woman: Sexual and Emotional Literacy for the Modern Man.* New York: Grove Press, 1986.

Stuart, Richard B., and Barbara Jacobson. *Weight, Sex, and Marriage: A Delicate Balance.* New York: Fireside, 1987.

Taylor, Jill M.; Gillian, Carol; and Amy M. Sullivan. *Between Voice and Silence: Women and Girls, Race and Relationship.* Cambridge, MA: Harvard University Press, 1995.

"Testosterone and the Heart." *Harvard Medical School Family Health Guide.* April 1, 2010. http://www.health.harvard.edu.

"Testosterone for Women." *Johns Hopkins: Health Alerts.* April 18, 2007. http://www.johnshopkinshealthalerts.com/.

"Testosterone Reference Ranges in Adults." *Quest Diagnostics.* December 2011. http://www.questdiagnostics.com/hcp/intguide/EndoMetab/Gen_Misc/Testosterone/Table%201.pdf.

Tisdale, Sallie. *Talk Dirty to Me: An Intimate Philosophy of Sex.* New York: Anchor Books, 1994.

Tokunaga, Adam. *Slow Sex Secrets: Lessons from the Master Masseur.* New York: Vertical, 2008.

Tolman, Deborah L. *Dilemmas of Desire: Teenage Girls Talk About Sexuality.* Cambridge, MA: Harvard University Press, 2002.

Weiner-Davis, Michele. *The Sex-Starved Marriage.* New York: Simon & Schuster, 2003.

Westman, Eric C.; Phinney, Stephen D.; and Jeff S. Volek. *The New Atkins for the New You: The Ultimate Diet for Shedding Weight and Feeling Great.* New York: Fireside, 2010.

Wills, S.; Ravipati, A.; Venuturumilli, P.; Kresge, C.; Folkerd, E.; Dowsett, M.; Hayes, D.; and D. Decker. "Effects of Vaginal Estrogens on Serum Estradiol Levels in Postmenopausal Breast Cancer Survivors Taking an Aromatase Inhibitor or a Selective Estrogen Receptor Modulator." *Cancer Research* 69 (2009): 806. doi: 10.1158/0008-5472.SABCS-09-806.

Wolf, Naomi. *The Beauty Myth.* New York: Harper Perennial, 2002.

Zoldbrod, Aline P. *Sex Smart: How Your Childhood Shaped Your Sexual Life and What to Do About It.* Oakland: New Harbinger Publications, 1998.